The Treatment of Myeloid Malignancies with Kinase Inhibitors

Editor

ANN MULLALLY

HEMATOLOGY/ONCOLOGY CLINICS OF NORTH AMERICA

www.hemonc.theclinics.com

Consulting Editors
GEORGE P. CANELLOS
H. FRANKLIN BUNN

August 2017 • Volume 31 • Number 4

ELSEVIER

1600 John F. Kennedy Boulevard • Suite 1800 • Philadelphia, Pennsylvania, 19103-2899

http://www.theclinics.com

HEMATOLOGY/ONCOLOGY CLINICS OF NORTH AMERICA Volume 31, Number 4
August 2017 ISSN 0889-8588, ISBN 13: 978-0-323-53235-8

Editor: Stacy Eastman
Developmental Editor: Kristen Helm

Hematology/Oncology Clinics (ISSN 0889-8588) is published bimonthly by Elsevier Inc., 360 Park Avenue South, New York, NY 10010-1710. Months of issue are February, April, June, August, October, and December. Business and Editorial Offices: 1600 John F. Kennedy Blvd., Ste. 1800, Philadelphia, PA 19103–2899. Customer Service Office: 3251 Riverport Lane, Maryland Heights, MO 63043. Periodicals postage paid at New York, NY and at additional mailing offices. Subscription prices are $397.00 per year (domestic individuals), $742.00 per year (domestic institutions), $100.00 per year (domestic students/residents), $453.00 per year (Canadian individuals), $919.00 per year (Canadian institutions) $536.00 per year (international individuals), $919.00 per year (international institutions), and $255.00 per year (international and Canadian students/residents). International air speed delivery is included in all *Clinics* subscription prices. All prices are subject to change without notice. **POSTMASTER:** Send address changes to *Hematology/Oncology Clinics of North America*, Elsevier Health Sciences Division, Subscription Customer Service, 3251 Riverport Lane, Maryland Heights, MO 63043. Customer Service (orders, claims, online, change of address): Elsevier Health Sciences Division, Subscription **Customer Service, 3251 Riverport Lane, Maryland Heights, MO 63043. Tel: 1-800-654-2452 (U.S. and Canada); 314-447-8871 (outside U.S. and Canada). Fax: 314-447-8029. E-mail: journalscustomerservice-usa@elsevier.com (for print support); journalsonlinesupport-usa@elsevier.com (for online support).**

Reprints. For copies of 100 or more, of articles in this publication, please contact the Commercial Reprints Department, Elsevier Inc., 360 Park Avenue South, New York, New York 10010-1710; Tel.: 212-633-3874, Fax: 212-633-3820, E-mail: reprints@elsevier.com.

Hematology/Oncology Clinics of North America is covered in *MEDLINE/PubMed (Index Medicus), EMBASE/ Excerpta Medica,* and *BIOSIS.*

Contributors

CONSULTING EDITORS

GEORGE P. CANELLOS, MD
William Rosenberg Professor of Medicine, Department of Medical Oncology, Dana-Farber Cancer Institute, Boston, Massachusetts

H. FRANKLIN BUNN, MD
Professor of Medicine, Division of Hematology, Brigham and Women's Hospital, Harvard Medical School, Boston, Massachusetts

EDITOR

ANN MULLALLY, MD
Assistant Professor of Medicine, Harvard Medical School, Division of Hematology, Brigham and Women's Hospital, Boston, Massachusetts

AUTHORS

OMAR ABDEL-WAHAB, MD
Human Oncology and Pathogenesis Program, Memorial Sloan Kettering Cancer Center, New York, New York

MICHAEL W. DEININGER, MD, PhD
Division of Hematology and Hematologic Malignancies, Huntsman Cancer Institute, The University of Utah, Salt Lake City, Utah

AHMET DOGAN, MD, PhD
Department of Pathology, Memorial Sloan Kettering Cancer Center, New York, New York

JACQUELINE S. GARCIA, MD
Instructor in Medicine, Department of Medical Oncology, Dana-Farber Cancer Institute, Harvard Medical School, Boston, Massachusetts

GABRIEL GHIAUR, MD, PhD
Adult Leukemia Program, Division of Hematological Malignancies, Sidney Kimmel Comprehensive Cancer Center, Assistant Professor of Oncology and Medicine, Johns Hopkins University, Baltimore, Maryland

JASON GOTLIB, MD, MS
Professor of Medicine (Hematology), Stanford Cancer Institute/Stanford University School of Medicine, Stanford, California

GABRIELA S. HOBBS, MD
Instructor in Medicine, Division of Hematology/Oncology, Massachusetts General Hospital, Harvard Medical School, Boston, Massachusetts

MARK LEVIS, MD, PhD
Adult Leukemia Program, Division of Hematological Malignancies, Sidney Kimmel
Comprehensive Cancer Center, Professor of Oncology and Medicine, Johns Hopkins
University, Baltimore, Maryland

JULIE-AURORE LOSMAN, MD, PhD
Assistant Professor, Department of Medical Oncology, Division of Hematology,
Dana-Farber Cancer Institute, Brigham and Women's Hospital, Harvard Medical School,
Boston, Massachusetts

MICHAEL J. MAURO, MD
Myeloproliferative Neoplasms Program, Leukemia Section, Memorial Sloan Kettering
Cancer Center, New York, New York

SARA C. MEYER, MD, PhD
Division of Hematology and Department of Biomedicine, University Hospital Basel, Basel,
Switzerland

ANN MULLALLY, MD
Assistant Professor of Medicine, Harvard Medical School, Division of Hematology,
Brigham and Women's Hospital, Boston, Massachusetts

THOMAS O'HARE, PhD
Division of Hematology and Hematologic Malignances, Huntsman Cancer Institute,
The University of Utah, Salt Lake City, Utah

NEVAL OZKAYA, MD
Department of Pathology, Memorial Sloan Kettering Cancer Center, New York, New York

AMI B. PATEL, MD
Huntsman Cancer Institute, The University of Utah, Salt Lake City, Utah

JERALD P. RADICH, MD
Clinical Research Division, Fred Hutchinson Cancer Research Center, Seattle,
Washington

SARAH ROZELLE, PhD
Division of Hematology, Department of Medicine, Brigham and Women's Hospital,
Harvard Medical School, Boston, Massachusetts

ROB SELLAR, MD
Postdoctoral Fellow, Division of Hematology, Brigham and Women's Hospital, Boston,
Massachusetts

RICHARD M. STONE, MD
Professor of Medicine, Department of Medical Oncology, Dana-Farber Cancer Institute,
Harvard Medical School, Boston, Massachusetts

JEFFREY W. TYNER, PhD
Associate Professor, Department of Cell, Developmental & Cancer Biology, Knight
Cancer Institute, Oregon Health & Science University, Portland, Oregon

Contents

Following the discovery of the JAK2V617F mutation, Janus kinase (JAK) 2 inhibitors were developed as rationally designed therapy in myeloproliferative neoplasms (MPNs). Although JAK2 inhibitors have clinical efficacy in MPN, they are not clonally selective for the JAK2V617F-mutant cells. Because activated JAK-signal transducer and activator of transcription (STAT) signaling is a common feature of MPN, JAK2 inhibitors are efficacious regardless of the specific MPN phenotypic driver mutation. The Food and Drug Administration approved the JAK1/JAK2 inhibitor, ruxolitinib, for the treatment of myelofibrosis and polycythemia vera. Additional JAK2 inhibitors are currently in advanced phased clinical trials.

Myeloproliferative neoplasms are driven by activated JAK2 signaling due to somatic mutations in JAK2, the thrombopoietin receptor MPL or the chaperone calreticulin in hematopoietic stem/progenitor cells. JAK2 inhibitors have been developed, but despite clinical benefits, they do not significantly reduce the mutant clone. Loss of response to JAK2 inhibitors occurs and several mechanisms of resistance, genetic and functional, have been identified. Resistance mutations have not been reported in MPN patients suggesting incomplete target inhibition. Alternative targeting of JAK2 by HSP90 inhibitors or type II JAK2 inhibition overcomes resistance to current JAK2 inhibitors. Additional combined therapy approaches are currently being evaluated.

The World Health Organization's semimolecular classification of eosinophilias emphasizes neoplasms driven by fusion tyrosine kinases. More than 80% of patients with systemic mastocytosis carry the KIT D816V mutation, the primary driver of disease pathogenesis. Genetic annotation of these diseases is critical and affords opportunities for targeted therapy. This article discusses our understanding of the mutated tyrosine kinome of eosinophilic neoplasms and systemic mast cell disease, and the successes and limitations of available therapies. Use of tyrosine kinase inhibitors as a bridge to hematopoietic stem cell transplantation, and development of more selective and potent tyrosine kinase inhibitors is also highlighted.

FLT3 mutations, generally associated with a poor prognosis, are found in approximately one-third of patients with acute myeloid leukemia (AML) and represent an attractive therapeutic target. FLT3 inhibitors undergoing clinical evaluation include first-generation relatively non-specific small molecules and second-generation compounds with higher potency and selectivity against mutant FLT3. Recently presented results from a prospective randomized clinical trial will likely lead to a change in the standard of care for younger patients with FLT3-mutated AML: addition of the multi-targeted FLT3 inhibitor midostaurin to standard induction and consolidation chemotherapy. Thus, personalized therapies for this subset of AML will soon be possible.

HEMATOLOGY/ONCOLOGY CLINICS OF NORTH AMERICA

THE CLINICS ARE AVAILABLE ONLINE!
Access your subscription at:
www.theclinics.com

Preface

Kinase Inhibitors in the Treatment of Myeloid Malignancies

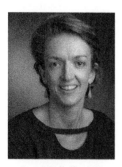

Ann Mullally, MD
Editor

Aberrant signaling pathway activation is a central feature of myeloid malignancies. With the development of the tyrosine kinase inhibitor, imatinib, to treat chronic myelogenous leukemia (CML), the paradigm of targeted therapy in cancer was established. Imatinib inhibits ABL, KIT, and platelet-derived growth factor receptor signaling and as a result is approved for the treatment of CML and subsets of patients with systemic mastocytosis (SM) and hypereosinophilic syndrome. Activated JAK-STAT signaling is central to the pathogenesis of *BCR-ABL*-negative myeloproliferative neoplasms (MPN), and the JAK1/2 inhibitor, ruxolitinib, is approved for the treatment of myelofibrosis and polycythemia vera. Most recently, midostaurin, a multikinase inhibitor with activity against FLT3 and KIT, was approved for the treatment of *FLT3*-mutant acute myeloid leukemia and advanced SM. In this issue, we present a series of reviews by leaders in the field, which describe the key research studies that led to the development and approval of these therapies and outline our current knowledge on mechanisms of resistance. We bookend these reviews with an article outlining key biological concepts underpinning the targeting of oncogenic kinases in myeloid malignancies and two articles describing some new developments in the field; the use of functional kinase inhibitor screens has uncovered novel therapeutic susceptibilities in myeloid blood cancers (eg, JAK inhibition in *CSF3R*-mutant chronic neutrophilic leukemia), and the application of genetic sequencing to histiocytic neoplasms has identified recurrent somatic mutations that activate mitogen-activated protein kinase signaling, which can be effectively targeted. We believe readers will find these reviews

Hematol Oncol Clin N Am 31 (2017) ix–x
http://dx.doi.org/10.1016/j.hoc.2017.05.001
0889-8588/17/© 2017 Published by Elsevier Inc.

hemonc.theclinics.com

informative and timely, providing a comprehensive overview of the current role of kinase inhibitors in the treatment of myeloid malignancies.

Ann Mullally, MD
Assistant Professor of Medicine
Harvard Medical School
Division of Hematology
Brigham and Women's Hospital
Harvard Institutes of Medicine Building
Room 738
77 Avenue Louis Pasteur
Boston, MA 02115, USA

E-mail address:
amullally@partners.org

Targeting Aberrant Signaling in Myeloid Malignancies: Promise Versus Reality

Rob Sellar, MD[a], Julie-Aurore Losman, MD, PhD[b],*

KEYWORDS

- Tyrosine kinase inhibitor • Acute myeloid leukemia • Myeloproliferative neoplasms
- BCR-ABL • JAK2 • Calreticulin • FLT3 • Oncogene addiction

KEY POINTS

- Clonal myeloid diseases include the myeloproliferative neoplasms: chronic myeloid leukemia (CML), polycythemia vera (PV), essential thrombocythemia (ET), primary myelofibrosis (PMF), chronic eosinophilic leukemia (CEL), and systemic mastocytosis (SM); and acute myeloid leukemia (AML).
- Clonal myeloid diseases have in common the mutational activation of cellular kinases that play an important role in driving aberrant cell proliferation.
- Therapeutic targeting of activated cellular kinases has had mixed results in the treatment of clonal myeloid disorders.
- The variability in efficacy of kinase-targeted therapies is due to several different factors, including the feasibility of kinase targeting, the on-target and off-target toxicity of kinase targeting, and the extent to which different clonal myeloid disorders are "addicted" to their activated kinases.

INTRODUCTION

Clonal myeloid diseases are a group of acquired hematopoietic stem cell disorders that are characterized by clonal proliferation of 1 or more myeloid cell lineages. Acute myeloid leukemia (AML) results from the uncontrolled proliferation of abnormal myeloid progenitor cells, whereas myeloproliferative neoplasms (MPN) are characterized by excessive production of mature blood cells: neutrophils (in chronic myeloid leukemia [CML]), erythrocytes (in polycythemia vera [PV]), megakaryocytes (in

Disclosure Statement: Nothing to disclose.
[a] Division of Hematology, Brigham and Women's Hospital, 1 Blackfan Circle, Karp Building, CHRB05.125, Boston, MA 02115, USA; [b] Department of Medical Oncology, Division of Hematology, Dana-Farber Cancer Institute, Brigham and Women's Hospital, Harvard Medical School, 450 Brookline Avenue, Boston, MA 02215, USA
* Corresponding author.
E-mail address: JulieAurore_Losman@dfci.harvard.edu

Hematol Oncol Clin N Am 31 (2017) 565–576
http://dx.doi.org/10.1016/j.hoc.2017.04.001
0889-8588/17/© 2017 Elsevier Inc. All rights reserved.

essential thrombocythemia [ET] and primary myelofibrosis [PMF]), eosinophils (in chronic eosinophilic leukemia [CEL]) and mast cells (in systemic mastocytosis [SM]).[1] Except in the case of PMF, cellular maturation in MPN proceeds normally and the expanded cell populations are functionally intact. In PMF, megakaryocyte differentiation is dysregulated and is thought to trigger the release of cytokines that, induce reactive bone marrow fibrosis and extramedullary hematopoiesis.[2] MPN and AML are driven by diverse genetic alterations but they have in common the mutational activation of cellular kinases, and dysregulated cytokine signaling has been found to play a key role in the pathophysiology of clonal myeloid disorders. This has provided a strong rationale for the therapeutic targeting of dysregulated kinase signaling to treat MPN and AML.

CML is emblematic of the promise of kinase inhibitors as anticancer therapy. CML is an indolent leukemia with a high rate of progression to "blast-phase CML," a highly aggressive acute leukemia with a particularly poor prognosis.[3] The genetic driver in CML is a fusion oncoprotein, BCR-ABL, that is the product of a balanced translocation between chromosomes 9 and 22 that gives rise to the "Philadelphia chromosome." BCR-ABL has constitutive Abelson (ABL) tyrosine kinase activity, and the proliferation and survival of CML cells is absolutely dependent on this kinase activity. This makes BCR-ABL's role in CML a paradigm of "oncogene addiction."[4] Because of their oncogene-addicted state, CML cells are exquisitely sensitive to tyrosine kinase inhibition, and tyrosine kinase inhibitors (TKI) have revolutionized the treatment of CML. A previously near-universally fatal malignancy has been transformed into a chronic disease with long-term remission rates of more than 90%.[5]

TKI therapy is the culmination of 4 decades of intensive laboratory investigation. The Philadelphia chromosome was discovered by Peter Nowell and David Hungerford in 1960.[6] This was followed by discovery of the t(9;22) chromosomal translocation by Janet Rowley in 1973,[7] characterization of the BCR-ABL fusion protein by Nora Heisterkamp and John Groffen in 1985,[8] confirmation of the in vitro oncogenic activity of BCR-ABL by Owen Witte in 1987,[9] and validation of the ability of BCR-ABL to induce CML in vivo by George Q. Daley and Richard Van Etten in 1999.[10] In 1996, Brian Druker and colleagues[11] identified a specific inhibitor of Abl kinase activity, CGP-57148, that selectively kills BCR-ABL–transformed cells. In 2001, CGP-57148, better known as imatinib, received accelerated Food and Drug Administration (FDA) approval for the treatment of CML.

The discovery of the Philadelphia chromosome in 1960 to the FDA approval of imatinib in 2001 took 40 years. In the modern era, this timeline has been dramatically shortened and the time from discovery of a genetic lesion to first-in-human clinical trials is steadily decreasing. For example, in 2005, the activating JAK2 mutation JAK2V617F was found to be highly recurrent in PV, ET, and PMF.[12] Just 6 years later, in 2011, the first-in-class JAK2 inhibitor, Ruxolitinib, was approved for use in patients.[13] Fig. 1 outlines the time from identification of specific clonal myeloid disease mutations to clinical targeting of the mutations in patients. This accelerated timeline reflects, in part, the fact that a number of previously developed drugs are being repurposed to target other oncogenic kinases. For example, Dasatinib, a TKI that was originally engineered to target BCR-ABL, was found to have in vitro activity against the stem cell factor receptor tyrosine kinase (KIT) mutation KITD816V, an imatinib-resistant activating mutation in KIT that is present in more than 80% of cases of SM.[14,15] Several other factors have contributed to this recent acceleration in target discovery and drug development, including large-scale sequencing efforts in cancer, improved technologies that allow for more rapid building of in vitro and in vivo models, and industrialized high-throughput compound screening.

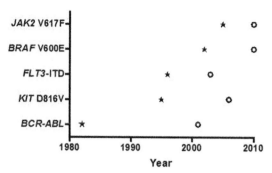

Fig. 1. The time from discovery of kinase mutations in clonal myeloid disorders (*stars*) to first-in-human clinical trials for kinase inhibitors (*open circles*) has progressively decreased over the past 3 decades.

Inspired by the success of TKIs in CML, laboratories around the world have for years been working to target other oncogenic enzymes in other cancers. Although there have been a number of notable success stories, including epidermal growth factor receptor (EGFR) inhibitors for the treatment of EGFR-mutant non–small-cell lung cancer (NSCLC),[16] BRAF and mitogen-activated protein kinase-kinase (MEK) inhibitors for the treatment of BRAF-mutant melanoma,[17] and anaplastic lymphoma kinase (ALK) inhibitors for the treatment of ALK-rearranged NSCLC,[18] none of these drugs has had the profound therapeutic efficacy of TKIs in CML. Even in other hematologic malignancies, targeted therapies have, for the most part, fallen short. JAK inhibitors in JAK2-mutant PV, ET, and PMF,[19,20] and FLT3 inhibitors in FLT3-mutant AML,[21,22] do have antidisease activity, but they have not been able to induce sustained remissions or to significantly prolong survival of patients with these diseases.

This introductory article explores reasons why, despite major advances in our understanding of the pathophysiology of clonal myeloid diseases, and despite the accelerated translation of biological findings into therapeutic agents, efforts to target oncogenic kinases in myeloid malignancies have been largely disappointing. We ask what lessons can be learned from these setbacks and discuss alternative therapeutic approaches that are currently being explored that may lead to more successful targeting of signaling pathways in clonal myeloid disorders and in cancer in general.

WHAT MAKES A GOOD DRUG-TARGET PAIRING?

TKIs have been successful in the treatment of CML for clearly identifiable reasons. First and foremost, the ABL kinase domain is highly amenable to drug targeting. Second, the pathways that are activated by BCR-ABL play an essential role in the pathophysiology of CML. Third, inhibition of ABL does not result in unacceptable toxicity. Several decades of work identifying, validating, and targeting oncogenic enzymes has taught us that, for a drug-target pairing to be truly successful, all 3 of these criteria must be met. Although this may seem, at first glance, to be a straightforward proposition, the reality is that these criteria set a very high bar for success that few drug-target pairings have, to date, been able to achieve.

DRUGGING THE UNDRUGGABLE

Not all cancer-associated activating mutations in signaling proteins are amenable to molecular targeting. A classic example is the RAS family of small GTPases. RAS

GTPases are among the most frequently mutated genes in cancer, and more than 10% of AML cases harbor activating RAS mutations.[23] Despite years of research, efforts to directly inhibit RAS have, to date, been unsuccessful.[24] One challenge to targeting RAS is structural. Unlike the ATP-binding domains of tyrosine kinases, which are structured pockets on the surface of the kinases that are amenable to small molecule targeting, the GTP-binding domains of RAS are not clearly defined structures to which small molecules can readily bind with high specificity and high affinity. Another challenge relates to the different mechanisms by which ATP and GTP modulate enzymatic activity. Tyrosine kinases bind ATP with low micromolar affinity and catalyze the rapid transfer of γ-phosphoryl groups from ATP to tyrosine residues on their substrates. This makes it possible for ATP-competitive inhibitors, such as imatinib, to effectively inhibit kinase activity in cells. RAS, on the other hand, binds GTP with picomolar affinity and cycles between a GTP-bound active state and a GDP-bound inactive state, making competitive inhibition of GTP binding to RAS unfeasible. Because of these biophysical constraints, efforts to target RAS have primarily focused on inhibiting functionally important posttranslational modifications of RAS and downstream effectors of RAS, rather than on directly inhibiting RAS itself. For example, the enzyme farnysyltransferase attaches a farnysyl moiety to RAS that facilitates its localization to the inner surface of the plasma membrane, and the membrane localization of RAS has been found to be required for its oncogenic activity.[25] Unfortunately, attempts to target farnysyltransferase in RAS-mutant clonal myeloid diseases have, so far, been disappointing, likely due to the existence of alternative RAS-activating posttranslational modifications, including geranylgeranylation.[26,27] Another strategy is to target RAS effector pathways. Inhibitors of phosphatidylinositol 3-kinase,[28] MEK,[29] and protein kinase B (AKT)[30] have all been found to have modest antileukemic activity in patients, and efforts to combine these therapies are currently ongoing. However, it is not known whether these drug combinations will be able to inhibit oncogenic RAS signaling sufficiently to induce durable remissions in patients and also have tolerable side-effect profiles.

ONCOGENE ADDICTION VERSUS DISEASE ACCELERATION

In 2014, 3 groups reported that a significant proportion of older individuals with normal blood counts harbor somatic mutations in their hematopoietic stem cell compartment in genes associated with hematologic malignancies.[31–33] This subclinical clonal hematopoiesis, termed clonal hematopoiesis of indeterminate potential (CHIP), is associated with an increased risk of developing hematologic malignancies. Prior studies on the mutational hierarchy of AML found that mutations in several epigenetic genes, including TET2, DNMT3A, and ASXL1, are likely to be early events in the clonal evolution of AML.[33,34] Interestingly, these same genes are the most frequently mutated in CHIP. Altogether, these observations suggest that CHIP-associated mutations are "founder mutations" that initiate clonal hematopoiesis, and that CHIP is a premalignant condition.

Interestingly, of the genes associated with CHIP, only JAK2 and CBL function through dysregulation of cytokine signaling. Mutations in other AML-associated kinases, including FLT3, KIT, and platelet-derived growth factor receptor, have not been found in CHIP, which is consistent with studies that suggest that kinase mutations are typically late events in clonal hematopoiesis.[35,36] This has profound therapeutic implications because even the most potent inhibitor of an oncogenic kinase can only inhibit the proliferation and survival of AML cells that are dependent on that kinase. If only a subset of a patient's malignant cells is dependent on a kinase, then inhibition of that kinase will leave any nonaddicted cells untouched, and the disease will persist. That is not to say that "late" mutational events are necessarily poor drug targets. If a mutant kinase were to drive a preleukemic clone to become fully transformed, then targeting that kinase could induce a durable clinical remission because the ancestral clone would need to acquire new mutations to mediate disease relapse. On the other hand, targeting a mutant kinase that simply accelerates the proliferation of already fully transformed cells is less likely to be effective. Inhibiting a kinase under these circumstances might eradicate the mutation-positive malignant clone and induce a transient clinical response, but it is unlikely to significantly alter the natural history of the disease.

Efforts to target FLT3 signaling in AML are illustrative of just how complex the interplay between a therapeutic target and its position in the clonal hierarchy of transformation can be. There are 2 major classes of *FLT3* mutations in AML, in-frame internal-tandem duplications in the juxtamembrane domain of FLT3, and point mutations in the tyrosine kinase domain of FLT3, both of which result in constitutive activation of FLT3 and activation of downstream signaling pathways.[37] Activating FLT3 mutations are typically late events in the clonal evolution of AML and are associated with increased white blood cell counts, high percentages of peripheral blood and bone marrow blasts, and poor overall survival. Several FLT3 inhibitors have been tested in patients, and response rates as high as 70% have been reported.[21,22] However, even patients treated with single-agent FLT3 inhibitors who experience a significant reduction in their blast count typically relapse within weeks, and FLT3 inhibitors have not significantly improved outcomes in patients with AML.

Despite the admittedly disappointing results of past clinical trials of FLT3 inhibitors, the specific characteristics of response and relapse in patients have been quite informative.[38] Multiple clinical trials have found a correlation between how potently FLT3 signaling is suppressed in a given patient and their likelihood of having a clinical response. This suggests that, in many patients, inhibiting FLT3 signaling does have antileukemic effects and FLT3 signaling does drive disease. Moreover, many patients with FLT3-mutant AML who initially respond to FLT3 inhibitors relapse with FLT3-mutant disease in which constitutive FLT3 signaling has been restored. This suggests that, in these patients, FLT3 inhibitors are acting "on-target" to drive selection for FLT3 inhibitor-resistance. It also suggests that, despite being a "late" event, activation of FLT3 plays a central role in the pathophysiology of FLT3-mutant AML. However, there are also patients with FLT3-mutant AML who initially respond to FLT3 inhibitor therapy but who then rapidly relapse with FLT3 wild-type disease. This suggests that, in these patients, FLT3 inhibitors are able to successfully suppress or even eradicate FLT3-mutant cells, and FLT3 inhibition selects for coexisting AML cells that do not harbor a FLT3 mutation. So where does this leave mutant FLT3 as a therapeutic target? Is there a way to anticipate the extent to which a given patient's AML is dependent on FLT3 signaling? Can we predict when FLT3 is truly driving disease and when it is merely favoring the clonal expansion of a specific AML subclone?

There is one additional finding from the FLT3 inhibitor clinical trials that adds yet another layer of complexity to the question of who should be treated with these agents. Several trials have found that therapeutic responses to FLT3 inhibitors are not restricted to patients with FLT3-mutant AML.[22,38] In fact, many patients with FLT3 wild-type AML have experienced significant, albeit transient, responses to FLT3 inhibitor therapy. These responses could be the result of "off-target" activities of FLT3 inhibitors against other oncogenic pathways. Alternatively, they could signify that wild-type FLT3 signaling plays a role in driving the proliferation and survival of AML cells irrespective of their FLT3 mutational status. If so, should all patients with

AML be treated with FLT3 inhibitors? Should the goal of FLT3 inhibitor therapy be complete suppression of both wild-type and mutant FLT3 signaling? How would such a therapy be tolerated from a toxicity standpoint? One clue to this last question may be gleaned from mouse models. Mice with complete genetic deletion of FLT3 have reduced numbers of B-cell precursors and defective dendritic cell function, and their hematopoietic stem cells have a decreased ability to reconstitute myelopoiesis after transplantation, but the mice have normal mature hematopoietic parameters and are otherwise healthy.[39] It is therefore conceivable that patients would tolerate potent suppression of FLT3 signaling without significant on-target adverse effects.

ON-TARGET TOXICITY AS A THERAPEUTIC LIABILITY

Dysregulated JAK2 activation is the most common molecular feature of BCR-ABL–negative MPN. More than 90% of PV cases and approximately 50% of ET and PMF cases harbor JAK2V617F mutations,[11] and most JAK2V617F-negative ET and PMF cases harbor mutations in either Calreticulin (CALR) or the thrombopoietin receptor (MPL),[40–42] both of which act to aberrantly activate JAK2 signaling. JAK2 activation appears to play a central role in the pathogenesis of BCR-ABL–negative MPN, and the observation that patients with CHIP frequently harbor isolated mutations in JAK2 suggests that JAK2V617F alone is sufficient to initiate clonal hematopoiesis. Based on these observations, one would expect that JAK2 inhibitors should be highly effective in the treatment of BCR-ABL–negative MPN. Indeed, JAK2 inhibitors have been found to improve blood counts, reduce splenomegaly, and alleviate constitutional symptoms in most patients with PV and PMF.[13,19,20] However, JAK2 inhibitors do not significantly reduce JAK2V617F allele burden or induce molecular remissions in patients with MPN. There are a few possible explanations for the inability of JAK2 inhibitors to recapitulate the success of TKIs in CML. One possibility is that aberrant JAK2 activation drives the clinical features of BCR-ABL–negative MPN, but is not required for the survival of MPN stem cells. In this scenario, one would have to assume either that the initiation, but not the maintenance, of clonal hematopoiesis is induced by aberrant JAK2 signaling; or that other, as yet unidentified, mutations in JAK2-mutant CHIP patients are the actual drivers of clonal hematopoiesis. Another possibility is that JAK2 is responsible for initiating and promulgating clonal hematopoiesis, but the degree to which JAK2 is being inhibited by existing JAK2 inhibitors is not sufficient to eradicate MPN stem cells. In support of this latter hypothesis, it has been reported that genetic deletion of JAK2 in hematopoietic stem cells from MPL-mutant mice results in a more profound reduction in ET symptoms than JAK2 inhibitor treatment, and also markedly reduces mutant allele burden.[43] This suggests that more potent JAK2 inhibitors may have better therapeutic efficacy in BCR-ABL–negative MPN.

JAK2 is absolutely required for hematopoiesis. Germline deletion of Jak2 in mice is embryonically lethal early during development due to a lack of hematopoiesis and, in adult mice, conditional deletion of Jak2 is associated with severe defects in hematopoietic stem cell function, impaired hematopoiesis, and reduced survival.[44,45] This suggests that there is an ongoing hematopoietic requirement for Jak2 throughout life. Although these findings suggest that complete loss of JAK2 activity may not be well-tolerated in patients, it is important to note that the pharmacokinetics of target inhibition by a drug are vastly different than that of complete genetic deletion. It is possible that a therapeutic window exists that would permit sufficient JAK2 inhibition to eradicate MPN stem cells without completely suppressing normal hematopoietic stem cell function. It is also important to note that adult Jak2-null mice have histologically normal hearts, kidneys, lungs, and brains,[45] which suggests that the on-target toxicity of JAK2 inhibitors may be limited to the hematopoietic compartment. Based on these and other findings, a new generation of more potent JAK2 inhibitors are currently in clinical development.

The JAK2 inhibitors that are currently in clinical use are not specific for JAK2V617F. They also target wild-type JAK2. Indeed, for JAK2 inhibitors to have utility in CALR-mutant and MPL-mutant MPN they would have to target wild-type JAK2. But what about JAK2V617F-specific inhibitors? It is likely that drugs that inhibit only mutant JAK2 would be less toxic than pan-JAK2 inhibitors. Is such an approach feasible? There is precedent for mutant-specific targeted therapies. One recent example is the first-in-class inhibitors of mutant isocitrate dehydrogenase (IDH). IDH mutations are present in 10% to 20% of cases of normal karyotype de novo AML,[46] where they function as important oncogenic drivers of disease.[47,48] Because wild-type IDH enzymes are ubiquitously expressed and play an important role in cellular metabolism, considerable effort has been expended to design mutant-specific inhibitors, and several IDH inhibitors currently in clinical development have approximately 200-fold higher activity against mutant than wild-type IDH enzymes.[48,49] Perhaps for this reason, these inhibitors are remarkably well-tolerated, and dose-limiting toxicity has not been a significant issue in patients. Similar efforts to develop JAK2V617F-specific inhibitors are currently under way.

The question of whether it is preferable to specifically target a mutant kinase or to target both the mutant kinase and its wild-type counterpart depends on several issues, including the degree to which inhibition of the wild-type enzyme induces dose-limiting on-target toxicity (eg, JAK2), the actual feasibility of specifically targeting the mutant protein, and, most importantly, the degree to which dependence on the target is specific to cancer cells that harbor the mutation (eg, FLT3). In cases like FLT3, although mutant-specific inhibitors may be better tolerated, decreased toxicity could come at the expense of clinical efficacy.

WHERE DO WE GO FROM HERE?

The example of TKIs for the treatment of CML provides an important proof-of-concept that therapeutic targeting of kinases can have profound clinical benefits, but numerous efforts to target other oncogenic kinases have been less successful. A pessimist might view these setbacks as evidence that BCR-ABL is a unique oncogenic kinase that is not representative of the role of kinase signaling in cancer. But as we have discussed here, there is mounting experimental and clinical evidence to suggest that, at least in some cases, more effective inhibition of kinase signaling may improve clinical outcomes. So how do we leverage the wealth of scientific and clinical knowledge gained over the past several decades to do a better job of targeting oncogenic kinases? There are several therapeutic strategies that are currently being explored to safely and effectively inhibit kinase signaling in cancer:

1. As discussed previously, mutant-specific kinase inhibitors have the potential to potently inhibit oncogenic kinases without incurring excessive toxicity from inhibition of their wild-type counterparts. JAK2V617F-specific inhibitors, for example, may be able to side-step much of the hematologic toxicity that would be expected of potent inhibition of JAK2 signaling.

2. Another therapeutic strategy that may improve patient outcomes is to use combinations of targeted therapies that inhibit different components of the same oncogenic pathway. In melanoma, for example, combination BRAF and MEK inhibition improves median progression-free survival in patients when compared with BRAF inhibition alone.[17] In addition to improving clinical efficacy, inhibiting

multiple components of the same oncogenic pathway may achieve robust pathway inhibition with only partial inhibition of each individual component of the pathway. This has the advantage of not only being more feasible from a drug-development standpoint, but may also be less toxic. Multitargeted therapy should also decrease the risk of developing therapy-resistant disease. Antiretroviral therapy for the treatment of human immunodeficiency virus has taught us that using drug cocktails that target multiple steps in the viral lifecycle (viral entry, viral fusion, reverse transcription, integration, viral replication, and viral assembly) not only increases remission rates but also decreases the risk of drug resistance. This is likely to also be true in cancer.

3. In addition to targeting multiple components of an oncogenic pathway, targeting the same oncoprotein in multiple ways may improve outcomes. In metastatic HER2-positive breast cancer, combined therapy with trastuzumab (an anti-HER2 monoclonal antibody that blocks activation of downstream signaling) and pertuzumab (an anti-HER2 monoclonal antibody that prevents dimerization with HER3) improves progression-free survival compared with trastuzumab monotherapy.[50] In acute promyelocytic leukemia (APL), all-trans retinoic acid (ATRA) activates RAR-α-mediated cellular differentiation and arsenic trioxide induces the degradation of PML-RARα and triggers apoptosis.[51,52] Although both drugs have activity against APL, the combination of ATRA and arsenic trioxide is superior to monotherapy with either drug alone.[53]

4. A promising novel approach to targeting oncoproteins has recently emerged from studies of lenalidomide, a phthalimide immunomodulatory drug that is used to treat multiple myeloma and del-5q myelodysplastic syndromes. In multiple myeloma, lenalidomide functions by binding to Ikaros transcription factors and inducing their ubiquitination and proteasomal degradation,[54,55] whereas in del-5q MDS, lenalidomide targets casein kinase 1α to the proteasome.[56] Efforts are currently under way to use phthalimide derivatives to recruit other oncoproteins to ubiquitin ligase complexes to induce their degradation.[57] This targeting strategy represents a powerful new approach to inhibiting oncoproteins, even oncoproteins that are currently considered "undruggable."

5. The approaches outlined previously focus on inhibiting oncogenic drivers and/or their downstream targets. An alternative to this approach is to identify and exploit tumor-specific vulnerabilities that are induced by oncogenic mutations, so-called "synthetic lethal" interations.[58] Synthetic lethality is a genetic principle wherein the combined effects of perturbing 2 genes results in a lethal phenotype, whereas perturbation of either gene alone has minimal effects on cellular fitness. For example, BRCA mutations promote oncogenesis by impairing DNA repair pathways that use homologous recombination. Although this leads to the accumulation of mutations that promote breast and ovarian cancer, BRCA mutations also sensitize tumor cells to pharmacologic inhibition of poly ADP ribose polymerase, an enzyme that is required for single-strand break repair of DNA. It is possible that unchecked cytokine signaling by mutant kinases likewise induces therapeutically targetable vulnerabilities in clonal myeloid disorders.

SUMMARY

Although the extraordinary success of targeting BCR-ABL in CML has not, until now, been recapitulated in other diseases, much has been learned from these failures that will inform future efforts to target kinase signaling. Advances in our understanding of how kinase signaling promotes cellular transformation, and the advent of novel treatment strategies, are reasons for renewed optimism that more effective targeting of signaling pathways is not only possible, but is likely to significantly improve outcomes in patients with clonal myeloid disorders and other cancers.

REFERENCES

1. Arber DA, Orazi A, Hasserjian R, et al. The 2016 revision to the World Health Organization classification of myeloid neoplasms and acute leukemia. Blood 2016; 127:2391–405.
2. Zahr AA, Salama ME, Carreau N, et al. Bone marrow fibrosis in myelofibrosis: pathogenesis, prognosis and targeted strategies. Haematologica 2016;101: 660–71.
3. Chereda B, Melo JV. Natural course and biology of CML. Ann Hematol 2015;94: S107–21.
4. Weinstein IB. Cancer. Addiction to oncogenes–the Achilles heal of cancer. Science 2002;297:63–4.
5. Druker BJ, Guilhot F, O'Brien SG, et al. Five-year follow-up of patients receiving imatinib for chronic myeloid leukemia. N Engl J Med 2006;355:2408–17.
6. Nowell PC, Hungerford DA. Chromosome studies on normal and leukemic human leukocytes. J Natl Cancer Inst 1960;25:85–109.
7. Rowley JD. Letter: a new consistent chromosomal abnormality in chronic myelogenous leukaemia identified by quinacrine fluorescence and Giemsa staining. Nature 1973;243:290–3.
8. Heisterkamp N, Stam K, Groffen J, et al. Structural organization of the bcr gene and its role in the Ph' translocation. Nature 1985;315:758–61.
9. McLaughlin J, Chianese E, Witte ON. In vitro transformation of immature hematopoietic cells by the P210 BCR/ABL oncogene product of the Philadelphia chromosome. Proc Natl Acad Sci U S A 1987;84:6558–62.
10. Li S, Ilaria RL, Million RP, et al. The P190, P210, and P230 forms of the BCR/ABL oncogene induce a similar chronic myeloid leukemia-like syndrome in mice but have different lymphoid leukemogenic activity. J Exp Med 1999;189:1399–412.
11. Druker BJ, Tamura S, Buchdunger E, et al. Effects of a selective inhibitor of the Abl tyrosine kinase on the growth of Bcr-Abl positive cells. Nat Med 1996;2: 561–6.
12. Levine RL, Wadleigh M, Cools J, et al. Activating mutation in the tyrosine kinase JAK2 in polycythemia vera, essential thrombocythemia, and myeloid metaplasia with myelofibrosis. Cancer Cell 2005;7:387–97.
13. Mascarenhas J, Hoffman R. Ruxolitinib: the first FDA approved therapy for the treatment of myelofibrosis. Clin Cancer Res 2012;18:3008–14.
14. Longley BJ, Metcalfe DD, Tharp M, et al. Activating and dominant inactivating c-KIT catalytic domain mutations in distinct clinical forms of human mastocytosis. Proc Natl Acad Sci U S A 1999;96:1609–14.
15. Schittenhelm MM, Shiraga S, Schroeder A, et al. Dasatinib (BMS-354825), a dual SRC/ABL kinase inhibitor, inhibits the kinase activity of wild-type, juxtamembrane, and activation loop mutant KIT isoforms associated with human malignancies. Cancer Res 2006;66:473–81.
16. Lynch TJ, Bell DW, Sordella R, et al. Activating mutations in the epidermal growth factor receptor underlying responsiveness of non-small-cell lung cancer to gefitinib. N Engl J Med 2004;350:2129–39.
17. Flaherty KT, Infante JR, Daud A, et al. Combined BRAF and MEK inhibition in melanoma with BRAF V600 mutations. N Engl J Med 2013;367:1694–703.

18. Kwak EL, Bang YJ, Camidge DR, et al. Anaplastic lymphoma kinase inhibition in non-small-cell lung cancer. N Engl J Med 2010;363:1693–703.

19. Harrison C, Kiladjian JJ, Al-Ali HK, et al. JAK inhibition with ruxolitinib versus best available therapy for myelofibrosis. N Engl J Med 2012;366:787–98.

20. Vannucchi AM, Kiladjian JJ, Griesshammer M, et al. Ruxolitinib versus standard therapy for the treatment of polycythemia vera. N Engl J Med 2015;372:426–35.

21. Smith BD, Levis M, Beran M, et al. Single-agent CEP-701, a novel FLT3 inhibitor, shows biologic and clinical activity in patients with relapsed or refractory acute myeloid leukemia. Blood 2004;103:3669–76.

22. Fischer T, Stone RM, Deangelo DJ, et al. Phase IIB trial of oral Midostaurin (PKC412), the FMS-like tyrosine kinase 3 receptor (FLT3) and multi-targeted kinase inhibitor, in patients with acute myeloid leukemia and high-risk myelodysplastic syndrome with either wild-type or mutated FLT3. J Clin Oncol 2010;28:4339–45.

23. Prior IA, Lewis PD, Mattos C. A comprehensive survey of Ras mutations in cancer. Cancer Res 2012;72:2457–67.

24. Cox AD, Fesik SW, Kimmelman AC, et al. Drugging the undruggable RAS: mission possible? Nat Rev Drug Discov 2014;13:828–51.

25. Casey PJ, Solski PA, Der CJ, et al. p21ras is modified by a farnesyl isoprenoid. Proc Natl Acad Sci U S A 1989;86:8323–7.

26. Kurzrock R, Albitar M, Cortes JE, et al. Phase II study of R115777, a farnesyl transferase inhibitor, in myelodysplastic syndrome. J Clin Oncol 2004;22:1287–92.

27. Ravoet C, Mineur P, Robin V, et al. Farnesyl transferase inhibitor (lonafarnib) in patients with myelodysplastic syndrome or secondary acute myeloid leukaemia: a phase II study. Ann Hematol 2008;87:881–5.

28. Ragon BK, Kantarjian H, Jabbour E, et al. Buparlisib, a PI3K inhibitor, demonstrates acceptable tolerability and preliminary activity in a phase I trial of patients with advanced leukemias. Am J Hematol 2017;92(1):7–11.

29. Jain N, Curran E, Iyengar NM, et al. Phase II study of the oral MEK inhibitor selumetinib in advanced acute myelogenous leukemia: a University of Chicago phase II consortium trial. Clin Cancer Res 2014;20:490–8.

30. Tibes R, McDonagh KT, Lekakis L, et al. Phase I study of the novel Cdc2/CDK1 and AKT inhibitor terameprocol in patients with advanced leukemias. Invest New Drugs 2015;33:389–96.

31. Genovese G, Kähler AK, Handsaker RE, et al. Clonal hematopoiesis and blood-cancer risk inferred from blood DNA sequence. N Engl J Med 2014;371:2477–87.

32. Jaiswal S, Fontanillas P, Flannick J, et al. Age-related clonal hematopoiesis associated with adverse outcomes. N Engl J Med 2014;371:2488–98.

33. Xie M, Lu C, Wang J, et al. Age-related mutations associated with clonal hematopoietic expansion and malignancies. Nat Med 2014;20:1472–8.

34. Ding L, Ley TJ, Larson DE, et al. Clonal evolution in relapsed acute myeloid leukaemia revealed by whole-genome sequencing. Nature 2012;481:506–10.

35. Shouval R, Shlush LI, Yehudai-Resheff S, et al. Single cell analysis exposes intra-tumor heterogeneity and suggests that FLT3-ITD is a late event in leukemogenesis. Exp Hematol 2014;42:457–63.

36. Jawhar M, Schwaab J, Schnittger S, et al. Molecular profiling of myeloid progenitor cells in multi-mutated advanced systemic mastocytosis identifies KIT D816V as a distinct and late event. Leukemia 2015;29:1115–22.

37. Grafone T, Palmisano M, Nicci C, et al. An overview on the role of FLT3-tyrosine kinase receptor in acute myeloid leukemia: biology and treatment. Oncol Rev 2012;17:64–74.
38. Wander SA, Levis MJ, Fathi AT. The evolving role of FLT3 inhibitors in acute myeloid leukemia: quizartinib and beyond. Ther Adv Hematol 2014;5:65–77.
39. Mackarehtschian K, Hardin JD, Moore KA, et al. Targeted disruption of the flk2/flt3 gene leads to deficiencies in primitive hematopoietic progenitors. Immunity 1995;3:147–61.
40. Klampfl T, Gisslinger H, Harutyunyan AS, et al. Somatic mutations of calreticulin in myeloproliferative neoplasms. N Engl J Med 2013;369:2379–90.
41. Nangalia J, Massie CE, Baxter EJ, et al. Somatic CALR mutations in myeloproliferative neoplasms with nonmutated JAK2. N Engl J Med 2013;369:2391–405.
42. Pikman Y, Lee BH, Mercher T, et al. MPLW515L is a novel somatic activating mutation in myelofibrosis with myeloid metaplasia. PLoS Med 2006;3:e270.
43. Bhagwat N, Koppikar P, Keller M, et al. Improved targeting of JAK2 leads to increased therapeutic efficacy in myeloproliferative neoplasms. Blood 2014;123:2075–83.
44. Neubauer H, Cumano A, Müller M, et al. Jak2 deficiency defines an essential developmental checkpoint in definitive hematopoiesis. Cell 1998;93:397–409.
45. Park SO, Wamsley HL, Bae K, et al. Conditional deletion of Jak2 reveals an essential role in hematopoiesis throughout mouse ontogeny: implications for Jak2 inhibition in humans. PLoS One 2013;8:1–13.
46. Mardis ER, Ding L, Dooling DJ, et al. Recurring mutations found by sequencing an acute myeloid leukemia genome. N Engl J Med 2009;361:1058–66.
47. Losman JA, Looper RE, Koivunen P, et al. (R)-2-hydroxyglutarate is sufficient to promote leukemogenesis and its effects are reversible. Science 2013;339:1621–5.
48. Wang F, Travins J, DeLaBarre B, et al. Targeted inhibition of mutant IDH2 in leukemia cells induces cellular differentiation. Science 2013;340:622–6.
49. Deng G, Shen J, Yin M, et al. Selective inhibition of mutant isocitrate dehydrogenase 1 (IDH1) via disruption of a metal binding network by an allosteric small molecule. J Biol Chem 2015;290:762–74.
50. Swain SM, Baselga J, Kim SB, et al. Pertuzumab, trastuzumab, and docetaxel in HER2-positive metastatic breast cancer. N Engl J Med 2015;372:724–34.
51. Breitman TR, Collins SJ, Keene BR. Terminal differentiation of human promyelocytic leukemic cells in primary culture in response to retinoic acid. Blood 1981;57:1000–4.
52. Chen GQ, Zhu J, Shi XG, et al. In vitro studies on cellular and molecular mechanisms of arsenic trioxide (As2O3) in the treatment of acute promyelocytic leukemia: As2O3 induces NB4 cell apoptosis with downregulation of Bcl-2 expression and modulation of PML-RAR alpha/PML proteins. Blood 1996;88:1052–61.
53. Burnett AK, Russell NH, Hills RK, et al. Arsenic trioxide and all-trans retinoic acid treatment for acute promyelocytic leukaemia in all risk groups (AML17): results of a randomised, controlled, phase 3 trial. Lancet Oncol 2015;16:1295–305.
54. Krönke J, Udeshi ND, Narla A, et al. Lenalidomide causes selective degradation of IKZF1 and IKZF3 in multiple myeloma cells. Science 2014;343:301–5.
55. Lu G, Middleton RE, Sun H, et al. The myeloma drug lenalidomide promotes the cereblon-dependent destruction of Ikaros proteins. Science 2014;343:305–9.
56. Krönke J, Fink EC, Hollenbach PW, et al. Lenalidomide induces ubiquitination and degradation of CK1α in del(5q) MDS. Nature 2015;523:183–8.

57. Winter GE, Buckley DL, Paulk J, et al. Drug development. Phthalimide conjugation as a strategy for in vivo target protein degradation. Science 2015;348: 1376–81.

58. Kaelin WG Jr. The concept of synthetic lethality in the context of anticancer therapy. Nat Rev Cancer 2005;5:687–98.

Tyrosine Kinase Inhibitor Treatment for Newly Diagnosed Chronic Myeloid Leukemia

 CrossMark

Jerald P. Radich, MD[a],*, Michael J. Mauro, MD[b]

KEYWORDS

- Chronic myeloid leukemia • Tyrosine kinase Inhibitor • Imatinib • BCR-ABL
- Molecular response

KEY POINTS

- Tyrosine kinase inhibitor (TKI) therapy has radically changed the natural history of chronic myeloid leukemia.
- "First-line" therapy with imatinib or the second-generation TKIs produce similar long-term survival results, with different early and "late" toxicities.
- Progression to advanced phase disease appears to be less frequent in patients treated with second-generation TKIs.
- Molecular monitoring of BCR-ABL is a powerful tool to document treatment response.
- Some patients with sustained deep molecular response can undergo TKI discontinuation under close monitoring and not relapse.

INTRODUCTION: A SHORT HISTORY OF THE DEVELOPMENT OF TYROSINE KINASE INHIBITOR THERAPY

Chronic myeloid leukemia (CML) is a myeloproliferative disorder marked by the increased proliferation of granulocytic cell lineage cells that retain the ability to differentiate. Nowell and Hungerford in 1960[1] described a small chromosome in metaphase preparations of marrow from patients with CML. This abnormal chromosome was dubbed the Philadelphia chromosome (the location of the investigators parent institution) and was later demonstrated to be the result of a translocation between chromosomes 9 and 22 [t(9;22)(q34;q11)].[2] The translocation results in the production of an abnormal BCR-ABL fusion protein, which is a constitutively

[a] Clinical Research Division, Fred Hutchinson Cancer Research Center, 1100 Fairview Avenue North, D4-100, Seattle, WA 98104, USA; [b] Myeloproliferative Neoplasms Program, Leukemia Section, Memorial Sloan Kettering Cancer Center, 1275 York Avenue (Between 67th and 68th street), New York, NY 10065, USA
* Corresponding author.
E-mail address: jradich@fredhutch.org

Hematol Oncol Clin N Am 31 (2017) 577–587
http://dx.doi.org/10.1016/j.hoc.2017.04.006
0889-8588/17/© 2017 Elsevier Inc. All rights reserved.

hemonc.theclinics.com

active cytoplasmic tyrosine kinase.[3,4] The Ph chromosome is found in myeloid, erythroid, megakaryocytic and B-lymphoid cells, suggesting that the original genetic lesion occurs in a stem cell.

The normal ABL protein is a nonreceptor tyrosine kinase with important roles in signal transduction and the regulation of cell growth.[5] The BCR-ABL protein, unlike normal ABL, is constitutively active and has increased kinase activity, leading to continuous activation of several cytoplasmic and nuclear signal transduction pathways including STAT, RAS, JUN, MYC, and phosphatidylinositol-3 kinase.[6] In experimental mouse systems, BCR-ABL causes myeloproliferative diseases similar to human CML, although chronic phase has been difficult to simulate.[7-9] In vitro studies show that BCR-ABL expression allows cells to become cytokine independent, protects them from apoptotic responses to DNA damage, and increases adhesion of hematopoietic cells to extracellular matrix proteins.[10-12]

The advent of tyrosine kinase inhibitor (TKI) therapy has fundamentally changed the approach of treating CML. The first TKI against BCR-ABL was imatinib mesylate (also known as STI571; Gleevec/Glivec). Imatinib is a small molecule inhibitor of several protein tyrosine kinases including the ABL tyrosine kinase, C-KIT, and PDGF. Imatinib was found to specifically inhibit or kill proliferating myeloid cell lines containing BCR-ABL *without effect on normal cells*.[13] This observation quickly led to a phase 1 trial in 1998 testing imatinib in patients with chronic phase CML who had failed interferon (IFN) -based therapy.[14] Of 54 patients who received oral doses of imatinib of 300 mg/d or more, a remarkable (at the time, *unbelievable*) 53 had a complete hematologic response, and cytogenetic responses were seen in 54% of cases. A second study of 58 patients with myeloid or lymphoid blast crisis CML (or Ph-positive ALL) showed partial/complete response in 60% to 70% of patients.[15] The toxicity profile of imatinib in these phase 1 studies was very encouraging, lying between the relatively benign hydroxyurea and the more problematic IFN. Nausea, edema, and muscle cramps occurred in roughly 50% of patients with diarrhea, vomiting, rash, and headache seen in about a third of cases.

Phase 1 results were then confirmed in phase 2 studies, and in 2001 imatinib was approved in the United States for chronic phase CML resistant to IFN as well as CML in accelerated or blast phases. Next came the substantial (N = 1106 patients) IRIS phase 3 study comparing imatinib to IFN plus cytarabine for newly diagnosed chronic phase CML.[16] At 12 months, complete cytogenetic remission (CCyR) was seen in ~70% of the imatinib-treated patients versus 7% with IFN and Ara-C therapy, and progression was seen in only 1.4% of the imatinib group compared with 10.3% of the IFN cases. Moreover, therapy crossovers for drug toxicity occurred in a mere 1% of imatinib-treated patients compared with 19% of IFN-treated patients. The study was closed early based on the outstanding efficacy advantage of imatinib. The superb short-term results were confirmed by a 5-year follow-up, where the overall survival of imatinib-treated patients was 89%, with progression to advanced phase disease in 7%.[17] Remarkably, nearly 70% of patients remained in CCyR at the 5-year mark.

Thus, the shape of CML was changed forever.

TKI therapy has revolutionized the treatment of CML, giving patients with chronic phase disease a near normal age-adjusted lifespan.[18] Given this success, CML will become a very prevalent oncologic diagnosis in the future, despite its relatively low incidence of roughly 5000 cases per year in the United States. Estimates in the United States are for a steady-state prevalence of CML of roughly 200,000 individuals rather than the pre-TKI level of ~25,000 individuals. Thus, it is important for the general oncologist to recognize and appreciate the special issues in diagnosing and caring for patients with CML in order to optimize their short- and long-term treatment responses. The following discussion is a succinct "top 10" of issues to consider when treating newly diagnosed CML.

HOW TO DIAGNOSE CHRONIC MYELOID LEUKEMIA

CML is diagnosed by a complete blood cell count with differential, a peripheral blood smear, examination for splenomegaly, and bone marrow aspiration with biopsy.[19] The definitive diagnosis of CML is based on the presence of the Ph chromosome (t[9;22]) and/or the BCR-ABL translocation. The Ph is analyzed by cytogenetic analysis of the bone marrow cells, which is essential at diagnosis because this will also reveal if there are additional cytogenetic lesions, which implies advanced phase disease (see later discussion). The BCR-ABL translocation can be probed in bone marrow or peripheral blood by reverse transcription polymerase chain reaction (RT-PCR) of the BCR-ABL chimeric messenger RNA (mRNA), or by fluorescence in situ hybridization probes for the BCR-ABL gene fusion.[20,21] Often debated, a bone marrow study at the diagnosis of CML is still thus essential and suggested to fully evaluate for features of advanced phase (accelerated phase or blast crisis) disease and to maximize the yield of cytogenetic testing to identify the Ph chromosome. In addition, baseline measurement (pretreatment) of BCR-ABL mRNA by RT-PCR allows for individualization of molecular response trajectory and kinetics, which is increasingly appreciated as complementary to standard response milestones.

CLINICAL AND PATHOLOGIC STAGING OF CHRONIC MYELOID LEUKEMIA

CML is divided into 3 phases (chronic, accelerated, and blast phases) based principally on the number of immature white blood cells (WBCs; myeloblasts) observed in the blood or bone marrow.[6] CML is usually diagnosed in the chronic phase, and this is marked by proliferation of primarily the myeloid element, with elevated WBCs in the periphery and by expansion of the myeloid series in the bone marrow. Patients with chronic-phase disease have fewer than 10% blasts, and cytogenetic testing reveals the presence of the Ph chromosome (t[9;22]) and no other clonal abnormalities.

There are various scoring systems that blend clinical and laboratory data to yield a prognostic score. These scoring systems include the Sokal, Hasford, and Eutos[22–24] prognostic scores, and each places patients into a low-, intermediate-, or high-risk group. Fortunately, aside from subtle differences in the laboratory and clinical characteristics used, all perform equally well. Online prognostic risk calculators are readily available (eg, http://www.mdcalc.com/sokal-index-cml/).

Surprisingly, there is no clear consensus as to the definition of accelerated and blast phase disease, and different classification systems use different blast cutoffs. The most common definitions of accelerated phase are listed in. It should be noted that the World Health Organization (WHO) criteria are more often used by pathologists than clinicians, and the WHO criteria are infrequently used in clinical trials.

As with the accelerated phase, the percentage of blast cells required for diagnosis of blast-phase disease differs according to the guidelines used. The WHO classification calls for at least 20%, whereas the National Comprehensive Cancer Network (NCCN) and European Leukemia Net (ELN) classification requires at least 30%.[14,16]

OUTCOME MEASURES WITH TYROSINE KINASE INHIBITOR TREATMENT OF CHRONIC MYELOID LEUKEMIA

The basic tools for monitoring patients are bone marrow cytogenetics for the Ph chromosome and peripheral blood RT-PCR for the BCR-ABL transcript. The goal is to reach sequential milestones of response; historically and currently a primary goal is achievement of a CCyR, defined as the absence of the Ph chromosome, among at least 20 evaluable bone marrow metaphases. Patients who achieve a CCyR are then routinely monitored by peripheral blood RT-PCR of BCR-ABL mRNA. The definitions of treatment response are in **Table 1**.

MONITORING OF TREATMENT RESPONSE

The monitoring guidelines of the NCCN and ELN are slightly different, but can be distilled into a few simple points.[20,21] First, cytogenetics should be performed until a CCyR is established. Generally, this means testing every 3 months. Once a CCyR is obtained, further cytogenetic testing is not needed unless the clinical/laboratory situation changes (such as an unexpected increase in the peripheral blood BCR-ABL). RT-PCR is performed on the peripheral blood every 3 months from diagnosis; once a major molecular response (MMR) is established, RT-PCR can be reduced to every 3 to 6 months. In addition to MMR, guidelines note and advise action based on achievement of or lack of "early molecular response" (EMR), where initial BCR-ABL transcript reduction is 1 log ($10\times$ lower) from initial pretreatment levels, or reduced to $\sim$10% on the international standard/scale (IS) using a median 100% IS starting level. EMR is ideal to occur by 3 months of therapy and should occur within the first 6 months of TKI treatment. Judging achievement of EMR is one of the main reasons to measure BCR-ABL transcripts at diagnosis (pretreatment) so as to not underestimate or overestimate the degree of reduction expected, allowing individualization for each patient.

It should be noted that a BCR-ABL of 1% roughly equates to the level of CCyR; some centers will use only RT-PCR to monitor patients (after the Ph has initially been confirmed to make the diagnosis), and only perform cytogenetics if the BCR-ABL is not falling appropriately, or if it increases after initially falling. Indeed, if CCyR or deeper remission has been achieved, the pretest probability of morphologic and cytogenetic evidence of the Ph chromosome is very small, and in the absence of blood count changes or other concerns, bone marrow studies in patients in deeper remission are not often needed.

An increase in BCR-ABL transcript levels by RT-PCR can be attributed to either the development of resistance or poor adherence to treatment.[25–27] Studies have shown that rates of compliance with imatinib treatment range from less than 25% up to 90%, and worse outcomes are associated with lower adherence rates. Significant degrees of molecular response include loss of MMR or any higher level; increase in BCR-ABL greater than 1% should trigger consideration of more full evaluation for mechanisms of

Table 1	
Definitions of treatment response	
Type of Response	**Definition**
Complete hematologic response (CHR)	Normal differential, WBC, platelets, absence of splenomegaly
Major cytogenetic response	0%–35% Ph + marrow metaphases
CCyR	0% Ph + marrow metaphases
MMR (3-log reduction)	BCR-ABL/ABL $\leq$ 0.1% IS
MR$^{4.0}$ (4-log reduction)	BCR-ABL/ABL $\leq$ 0.01% (IS)
MR$^{4.5}$ (4.5-log reduction)	BCR-ABL/ABL $\leq$ 0.003% (IS)
CMR	Undetectable BCR-ABL (test of sensitivity $\geq$ 4.5 logs)

resistance, that is, bone marrow studies to rule out cytogenetic evolution or other features (**Table 2**).

INITIAL TYROSINE KINASE INHIBITOR THERAPY FOR CHRONIC PHASE CHRONIC MYELOID LEUKEMIA

The choices are imatinib, and the more potent second-generation TKIs nilotinib and dasatinib. Several randomized trials consistently show that the second-generation agents yield superior short-term responses (3–6 month molecular response, 12 month CCyR, and 12 month MMR), lower progression to advanced phase disease, but surprising similar overall survival to imatinib[15–17] (**Table 3**).

How do you pick one TKI over another for a newly diagnosed CML patient? Some basic considerations include *first:* what are the treatment goals? For an older patient, a reasonable goal is to control the disease with a bias toward a low risk of toxicity. In a younger patient, the goal can be to achieve a deeper molecular response with a hope for eventual discontinuation of TKI therapy (see later discussion,). *Second,* consideration of comorbidities should be undertaken. For example, it may be best to avoid nilotinib in a patient with active cardiovascular disease (see later discussion). *Third,* consider the disease status at the time of diagnosis; patients at low risk of progression (low Sokal/Hasford/Eutos score) may do well on imatinib, whereas patients with high-risk disease might benefit from the more potent second-generation TKIs. *Last,* personal experience and comfort level of the physician managing various side effects of specific TKIs remain crucial in the decision making process.

There have been multiple phase 2 trials, and 3 phase 3 trials demonstrating the superior short-term (12 months) efficacy of the second-generation TKI nilotinib and dasatinib over imatinib. Three separate randomized trials showed that nilotinib or dasatinib yielded more frequent CCyR and MMR by 12 months as well as fewer progressions to accelerated or blast phase, compared with imatinib.[28–30] However, these trials have failed to show a benefit in overall survival for nilotinib or dasatinib over imatinib.

CLINICALLY RELEVANT RESPONSE MILESTONES IN CHRONIC MYELOID LEUKEMIA TREATMENT

Most patients with chronic phase do very well on TKI therapy. However, patients who progress to advanced phase disease (accelerated and blast phases) are unlikely to

Table 2
Monitoring guidelines on tyrosine kinase inhibitor therapy

Test	Monitoring Guidelines
Cytogenetics (bone marrow)	• At diagnosis to establish disease phase • Every 3 mo until CCyR if PCR not available
BCR-ABL (peripheral blood)	• At diagnosis • Every 3 mo for 2 y and every 3–6 mo thereafter
Screen for ABL mutation (bone marrow or peripheral blood)	• Failure to reach NCCN/ELN treatment milestones • Any sign of loss of response • 1-log increase in *BCR-ABL* transcript levels and loss of MMR • Disease progression to accelerated or blast phase

Table 3
Responses of front-line tyrosine kinase inhibitor in chronic phase chronic myeloid leukemia

Outcome (%)	Imatinib	Dasatinib	Nilotinib
Discontinue	40–50	40	40
CCyR	60–70	70–80	70–80
MMR	50–60	70–80	70–80
Progression AP/BC	5–7	3–5	3–5
Overall survival	90–95	90–95	90–95

Abbreviation: AP/BC, accelerated phase/blast crisis.

achieve a stable/deep remission on a TKI, and their best bet is allogeneic stem cell transplant. Thus, it is paramount to monitor patients carefully and identify those cases who fail to hit response benchmarks. Based on many clinical studies, the NCCN and ELN have established treatment guidelines that include response milestones. Failure to achieve these milestones yield inferior short- and long-term outcomes compared with patients who reach the milestones. The NCCN and ELN guidelines are slightly different, but **Table 4** reflect the common elements of treatment failure.

MUTATIONAL ANALYSIS FOR RESISTANCE/RELAPSE

In roughly 50% of cases of TKI resistance, single base-pair mutations in the tyrosine binding domain of ABL are found. BCR-ABL kinase domain point mutations are associated with both imatinib resistance and secondary resistance. At least 100 different point mutations have been identified thus far. Thus, BCR-ABL kinase domain mutational analysis should be performed for all patients who do not hit the response milestones, or reach these milestones and then relapse. This population includes patients with disease that has progressed to the accelerated or blast phase as well as patients in the chronic phase who have an inadequate initial response to TKI therapy, loss of hematologic response or cytogenetic relapse, or a 1-log increase in BCR-ABL transcripts with a loss of MMR. Identification of the point mutation at the time of treatment failure is essential for determining the appropriate salvage therapy; second-line and third-line treatment options should be chosen based on the known effectiveness of a specific TKI for a specific point mutation.[31,32] Mutation testing at diagnosis, although common in other cancers, does not provide information to guide treatment and is not currently recommended, except in the case of new diagnosis in advanced phase of CML.

SWITCHING TO A DIFFERENT TYROSINE KINASE INHIBITOR FOR RESISTANCE

There are now 4 "next generation" TKIs approved for resistant chronic phase CML: nilotinib, dasatinib, bosutinib (second generation), and ponatinib (third generation). If

Table 4
When to switch frontline tyrosine kinase inhibitor therapy in chronic myeloid leukemia

Time	Definition of Failure to TKI
3 mo	No CHR, >95% Ph, and/or BCR-ABL >10% IS
6 mo	>35% Ph, and/or BCR-ABL >10% IS
12 mo	Ph> 0% and/or BCR-ABL > 1% IS
Any time point	Loss of CHR, CCyR, MMR, new clonal cytogenetic changes

a patient needs to change from imatinib, it makes sense to switch to a second-generation TKI; if a patient needs to switch from initial therapy with a second-generation therapy, then switching to another TKI is justified, but in general changing to a less potent TKI or an agent with greater chance of further resistance (ie, imatinib) is probably not the best option, and careful consideration of a third-generation agent (eg, ponatinib) for high-level resistance to initial therapy with a second-generation agent.

The same criterion considered for initial therapy choice applies to the choice of later lines of therapy as well. Consideration needs to be taken regarding specific side effect profiles, comorbidities of the patient, and physician and patient comfort level with a given TKI. However, the more important considerations in the face of resistance may be the disease state (chronic vs advanced) and the presence or absence of ABL point mutations, to decide the best course of action. There are hundreds of possible point mutations, but the most common have had in vitro testing performed, and ample literature exists showing which particular mutation is sensitive to a specific TKI. Ponatinib is unique among these agents, because it is the only TKI effective in patients with the T315I mutation. Moreover, it seems to be effective across the entire range of known ABL mutations. Time will tell if it becomes the first choice for resistant disease. The T315I mutation is seen in 4% to 15% of patients with imatinib resistance.[20,21] Other mutations of note include T315A, V299L, and F359V, which are associated with resistance to dasatinib, and Y253H, E255K/V, L273M, and F359V, which are associated with resistance to nilotinib.

TYROSINE KINASE INHIBITOR TOXICITY AND WHAT TO DO ABOUT IT

When there was only imatinib, all efforts were aimed to try to keep patients on the drug in the face of side effects. Now that there are a total of 5 US Food and Drug Administration–approved TKIs, the better course in patients with any toxicity that fosters poor adherence, dose reduction, or even drug discontinuation is to simply switch TKIs. Fortunately, the available agents appear to be generally "cross-tolerant"; that is, if a patient has a particular side effect on one TKI, he/she is relatively unlikely to have it on another TKI. One exception to this rule may be myelosuppression, which may be proportionally more related to disease and time on treatment than the specific TKI. The heterogeneity of toxicity and cross-tolerance may be to genetic polymorphisms in normal tissue and the different spectrum of kinases being targeted. Because CML is often diagnosed with a relative absence of symptoms, patients may actually feel worse taking a TKI than they did before they were diagnosed. This situation is a recipe for poor adherence, and several studies have demonstrated a shockingly poor compliance to the scheduled dosing of the TKIs, and is especially problematic because adherence is strongly associated with the ability to achieve important endpoints such as MMR and complete molecular response (CMR, see later discussion).

Common side effects of TKIs are noted in **Table 5**. Complete guides to symptom management can be found on the NCCN CML Guidelines web site (https://www.nccn.org). Of particular note is the need to be aware of longer term, or "late" complications from TKIs, especially cardiovascular and cardiopulmonary events. Serious vascular events, including myocardial infarction, cerebrovascular accident, and peripheral arterial occlusion, have been observed, as well as several symptoms suggestive of active vascular disease during TKI therapy. Dasatinib, even years after initiation, can continue to trigger pleural/pericardial fluid accumulation and symptoms; pulmonary hypertension is a more rare complication (<1%) but may also occur late into treatment. Nilotinib and ponatinib both have increased risk of vascular occlusive events, greater with ponatinib than any other TKI; dasatinib and bosutinib appear to have

Table 5
Considerations on tyrosine kinase inhibitor selection in chronic phase chronic myeloid leukemia

TKI	Advantage	Disadvantage
Imatinib	Long-term safety data Less expensive (generic)	Lower rates of CCyR, MMR compared with second-generation TKIs Fluid retention Gastrointestinal toxicity Musculoskeletal aches & pains
Dasatinib	>10% higher CCyR rate compared with Imatinib ~2× higher rates of MMR	Pleural effusion Pulmonary arterial hypertension Thrombocytopenia Hemorrhage
Nilotinib	>10% higher CCyR compared with Imatinib ~2× higher rates of MMR	Cumbersome dosing schedule Skin rash Pancreatitis QT prolongation Dyslipidemia/hyperglycemia Peripheral arterial disease/vascular occlusive disease

minimal vascular occlusive risk, and imatinib appears to have no clear vascular disease "signal" and may be either neutral or potentially protective. Although metabolic changes are seen with nilotinib (hyperglycemia, dyslipidemia), and hypertension is observed with ponatinib, the mechanism of these events remains poorly understood. Moreover, the mechanism of vascular occlusion has not been elucidated for any of the TKIs, and risk mitigation remains a challenge. Recommendations for monitoring for such events are emerging,[33] and age appropriate risk investigation, reduction, and event management irrespective of the CML status or drug, and increased surveillance if higher-risk TKIs are used, are the best approach at present. An emerging specialty within cardiology, cardio-oncology, is expected to provide increasing insight and capacity to monitor cardiovascular risk in cancer therapy patients, and referral to such subspecialists may be of great benefit in the long-term monitoring of CML patients.

DISCONTINUATION OF TYROSINE KINASE INHIBITOR AFTER PROLONGED "DEEP" MOLECULAR RESPONSE

It was first thought that patients would need to stay on TKIs forever, because in vitro work showed the putative CML stem cell survived in the presence of BCR-ABL inhibition. However, several studies have shown that approximately 40% patients who are in a CMR can successfully discontinue TKI therapy, and stay in CMR for several years.[33] Most patients relapse within 6 months after discontinuation, and so far, all patients have responded when rechallenged with a TKI, although not all have returned to CMR.

Given that the long-term consequences of TKI discontinuation are not known, the standard recommendation is that it should only be performed in the context of a clinical trial. However, in reality, the momentum toward discontinuation is rising in the nonacademic community, and to face this reality, the NCCN has listed a minimum set of criteria that one must have to consider discontinuation outside of a clinical trial. The key elements of CMR consideration include not only proper vetting of CML treatment response but continual short interval access to sensitive molecular testing and full disclosure and consent of the patient regarding the logistics, risk, and re-treatment requirements should TKI discontinuation prove unsuccessful.

SUMMARY

Primary therapy for chronic phase CML is extremely effective. Adherence to therapy and vigilant monitoring should keep resistance and progression to a minimum. However, resistance is not futile and can be treated with logical selection of "second-line" TKIs as well as allogeneic stem cell transplantation, if salvage therapy is unsuccessful. These topics will be considered in a later article in this collection.

REFERENCES

1. Nowell PC, Hungerford DA. A minute chromosome in human granulocytic leukemia. Science 1960;132:1497.
2. Rowley JD. A new consistent chromosomal abnormality in chronic myelogenous leukaemia identified by quinacrine fluorescence and Giemsa staining. Nature 1973;243(5405):290–3.
3. Faderl S, Talpaz M, Estrov Z, et al. The biology of chronic myeloid leukaemia. N Engl J Med 1999;341(3):164–72.
4. Naka K, Hoshii T, Tadokoro Y, et al. Molecular pathology of tumor-initiating cells: lessons from Philadelphia chromosome-positive leukaemia. Pathol Int 2011;61(9): 501–8.
5. Sawyers CL. Chronic myeloid leukemia. N Engl J Med 1999;340:1330–40 [Review].
6. McLaughlin J, Chianese E, Witte ON. In vitro transformation of immature hematopoietic cells by the P210 BCR/ABL oncogene product of the Philadelphia chromosome. Proc Natl Acad Sci U S A 1987;84:6558–62.
7. Heisterkamp N, Jenster G, ten Hoeve J, et al. Acute leukaemia in BCR/ABL transgenic mice. Nature 1990;344:251–3.
8. Daley GQ, van Etten RA, Baltimore D. Induction of chronic myelogenous leukemia in mice by the p210 BCR/ABL gene of the Philadelphia chromosome. Science 1990;247:824–30.
9. Kelliher MA, McLaughlin J, Witte ON, et al. Induction of a chronic myelogenous leukemia-like syndrome in mice with v-abl and BCR/ABL. Proc Natl Acad Sci U S A 1990;87:6649–53 [Erratum appears in Proc Natl Acad Sci U S A 1990;87:9072.].
10. Evans CA, Owen-Lynch PJ, Whetton AD, et al. Activation of the Abelson tyrosine kinase activity is associated with suppression of apoptosis in hemopoietic cells. Cancer Res 1993;53:1735–8.
11. Bazzoni G, Carlesso N, Griffin JD, et al. Bcr/Abl expression stimulates integrin function in hematopoietic cell lines. J Clin Invest 1996;98:521–8.
12. Wang JY. Abl tyrosine kinase in signal transduction and cell-cycle regulation. Curr Opin Genet Dev 1993;3:35–43 [Review].
13. Druker BJ, Tamura S, Buchdunger E, et al. Effects of a selective inhibitor of the Abl tyrosine kinase on the growth of Bcr-Abl positive cells. Nat Med 1996;2: 561–6.
14. Druker BJ, Talpaz M, Resta DJ, et al. Efficacy and safety of a specific inhibitor of the BCR-ABL tyrosine kinase in chronic myeloid leukemia. N Engl J Med 2001; 344:1031–7.

15. Druker BJ, Sawyers CL, Kantarjian H, et al. Activity of a specific inhibitor of the BCR-ABL tyrosine kinase in the blast crisis of chronic myeloid leukemia and acute lymphoblastic leukemia with the Philadelphia chromosome. N Engl J Med 2001; 344:1038–42.

16. O'Brien SG, Guilhhot F, Larson RA, et al. Imatinib compared with interferon and low-dose cytarabine for newly diagnosed chronic-phase chronic myeloid leukemia. N Engl J Med 2003;328:994–1004.

17. Druker BJ, Guilhot F, O'Brien SG, et al. Five-year follow-up of patients receiving imatinib for chronic myeloid leukemia. N Engl J Med 2006;355:2408–17.

18. Huang X, Cortes J, Kantarjian H. Estimations of the increasing prevalence and plateau prevalence of chronic myeloid leukemia in the era of tyrosine kinase inhibitor therapy. Cancer 2012;118(12):3123–7.

19. Vardiman JW, Harris NL, Brunning RD. The World Health Organization (WHO) classification of the myeloid neoplasms. Blood 2002;100(7):2292–302.

20. Version 3.2014NCCN clinical practice guidelines in oncology. Chronic myelogenous leukemia. National Comprehensive Cancer Network; 2014. Available at: http://www.nccn.org/professionals/physician_gls/pdf/cml.pdf. Accessed June 4, 2014.

21. Baccarani M, Deininger MW, Rosti G, et al. European LeukemiaNet recommendations for the management of chronic myeloid leukemia: 2013. Blood 2013;122(6): 872–84.

22. Sokal JE, Cox EB, Baccarani M, et al. Prognostic discrimination in "good-risk" chronic granulocytic leukemia. Blood 1984;63(4):789–99.

23. Hasford J, Pfirrmann M, Hehlmann R, et al. A new prognostic score for survival of patients with chronic myeloid leukemia treated with interferon alfa: Writing Committee for the Collaborative CML Prognostic Factors Project Group. J Natl Cancer Inst 1998;90(11):850–8.

24. Hasford J, Baccarani M, Hoffmann V, et al. Predicting complete cytogenetic response and subsequent progression-free survival in 2060 patients with CML on imatinib treatment: the EUTOS score. Blood 2011;118(3):686–92.

25. Marin D, Bazeos A, Mahon FX, et al. Adherence is the critical factor for achieving molecular responses in patients with chronic myeloid leukaemia who achieve complete cytogenetic responses on imatinib. J Clin Oncol 2010;28(14):2381–8.

26. Darkow T, Henk HJ, Thomas SK, et al. Treatment interruptions and non-adherence with imatinib and associated healthcare costs: a retrospective analysis among managed care patients with chronic myelogenous leukaemia. Pharmacoeconomics 2007;25(6):481–96.

27. Noens L, van Lierde MA, De Bock R, et al. Prevalence, determinants, and outcomes of nonadherence to imatinib therapy in patients with chronic myeloid leukaemia: the ADAGIO study. Blood 2009;113(22):5401–11.

28. Saglio G, Kim DW, Issaragrisil S, et al. Nilotinib versus imatinib for newly diagnosed chronic myeloid leukemia. N Engl J Med 2010;362(24):2251–9.

29. Kantarjian H, Shah NP, Hochhaus A, et al. Dasatinib versus imatinib in newly diagnosed chronic-phase chronic myeloid leukemia. N Engl J Med 2010; 362(24):2260–70.

30. Radich JP, Kopecky KJ, Appelbaum FR, et al. A randomized trial of dasatinib 100 mg versus imatinib 400 mg in newly diagnosed chronic-phase chronic myeloid leukemia. Blood 2012;120(19):3898–905.

31. Jabbour E, Jones D, Kantarjian HM, et al. Long-term outcome of patients with chronic myeloid leukaemia treated with second-generation tyrosine kinase

inhibitors after imatinib failure is predicted by the in vitro sensitivity of BCR-ABL kinase domain mutations. Blood 2009;114(10):2037–43.

32. Moslehi JJ, Deininger MW. Tyrosine kinase inhibitor-associated cardiovascular toxicity in chronic myeloid leukemia. J Clin Oncol 2015;33(35):4210–8.

33. Mahon FX, Réa D, Guilhot J, et al. Discontinuation of imatinib in patients with chronic myeloid leukaemia who have maintained complete molecular remission for at least 2 years: the prospective, multicentre Stop Imatinib (STIM) trial. Lancet Oncol 2010;11(11):1029–35.

Mechanisms of Resistance to ABL Kinase Inhibition in Chronic Myeloid Leukemia and the Development of Next Generation ABL Kinase Inhibitors

(R) CrossMark

Ami B. Patel, MD[a], Thomas O'Hare, PhD[b],
Michael W. Deininger, MD, PhD[b],*

KEYWORDS

- Chronic myeloid leukemia (CML) • Tyrosine kinase inhibitor (TKI) • BCR-ABL1
- Treatment-free remission (TFR) • Drug resistance • Mutation

KEY POINTS

- More than 25% of patients with chronic myeloid leukemia (CML) will switch tyrosine kinase inhibitors (TKIs) during their lifetime owing to resistance or intolerance.
- Ponatinib is the only TKI effective against the T315I BCR-ABL1 mutation; its activity derives from its lack of dependence on forming a critical hydrogen bond with residue T315 for high-affinity binding to BCR-ABL1.
- Diverse pathways involving growth factors, epigenetic regulators, and apoptotic machinery have been implicated in BCR-ABL1–independent resistance.
- CML leukemic stem cells are resistant to TKI therapy and contribute to minimal residual disease. Combination strategies using TKIs and other drugs are an intense focus of investigation.
- A minority of patients with CML who achieve sustained deep molecular responses on TKI therapy are able to discontinue treatment without molecular recurrence, entering a state called "treatment-free remission."

Disclosures: M.W. Deininger and T. O' Hare are supported by the NIH (1R01CA178397-01 and 1R21CA205936-01), V Foundation for Cancer Research, Hope Foundation, and University of Utah seed funding.
[a] Department of Hematology and Oncology, Huntsman Cancer Institute, 2000 Circle of Hope Drive, The University of Utah, Salt Lake City, UT 84112, USA; [b] Division of Hematology and Hematologic Malignancies, Huntsman Cancer Institute, The University of Utah, 2000 Circle of Hope Drive, Salt Lake City, UT 84112, USA
* Corresponding author.
E-mail address: Michael.deininger@hci.utah.edu

INTRODUCTION

Every year, more than 8000 new cases of chronic myeloid leukemia (CML) are diagnosed in the United States.[1] BCR-ABL1, a fusion protein kinase derived from a reciprocal translocation between chromosomes 9 and 22, is necessary and sufficient for CML pathogenesis.[2] Tyrosine kinase inhibitors (TKIs) of BCR-ABL1 have revolutionized CML therapy, with life expectancy now close to that of the general population.[3] As a result, the prevalence of CML is increasing, as patients on TKIs live with what is more and more viewed as a chronic ailment rather than a potentially lethal disease. It is estimated that more than 25% of patients with CML will switch TKIs at least once during their lifetime owing to TKI intolerance or resistance.[4] Mutations in the kinase domain (KD) of BCR-ABL1 are the most extensively studied mechanism of TKI resistance in CML, but fail to explain anywhere from 20% to 40% of resistant cases. Activation of alternative, BCR-ABL1–independent survival pathways has been implicated mechanistically in these cases, and may also explain the phenomenon of persistence in responding patients who fail to clear minimal residual disease (MRD) or experience recurrence upon discontinuation of therapy despite achieving deep molecular response (DMR, BCR-ABL1 $\leq$ 0.01% on the international scale).

DEFINITIONS

The National Comprehensive Cancer Network and the 2013 European LeukemiaNet guidelines recommend cytogenetic and/or molecular monitoring at 3, 6, and 12 months into frontline TKI therapy.[5,6] European LeukemiaNet recommendations categorize the molecular and cytogenetic responses at each time interval as "optimal," "warning," or "failure." Optimal responses are associated with a life expectancy similar to that of the general population, whereas failure is associated with TKI resistance and increased risk of disease progression or death, necessitating a change in TKI therapy. Failure to achieve complete hematologic response (normalization of peripheral blood counts, and resolution of splenomegaly and CML-related symptoms) or complete cytogenetic response (CCyR; 0% Ph$^+$ metaphases based on analysis of 20 bone marrow cells) within an allocated duration of time constitutes TKI failure, as does loss of these milestones or progression to accelerated phase or blastic phase at any time point. Whether failure to achieve major molecular response (MMR; BCR-ABL1 $\leq$ 0.1% on the international scale) in patients with CCyR defines failure is subject to ongoing debate. Similarly, confirmed loss of MMR while CCyR is maintained does not technically constitute failure, although most of these patients will go on to lose CCyR.[7]

Overt resistance such as loss of complete hematologic response or even progression to accelerated phase/BC-CML is associated with unfavorable clinical outcomes and represents a situation very different from persistent low-level disease associated with MRD, which is clinically relevant only in the context of TKI discontinuation. Primary resistance implies failure to achieve time-dependent endpoints of complete hematologic response, CCyR, and MMR upon initiation of TKI therapy, whereas secondary (acquired) resistance is defined as the loss of response.[8] At the mechanistic level, we classify TKI resistance as either BCR-ABL1 dependent or BCR-ABL1 independent (**Fig. 1**). Although this distinction seems formalistic, it does have a great degree of clinical relevance, because it informs the strategy required to combat resistance: BCR-ABL1-dependent resistance relies on mechanisms that subvert effective BCR-ABL1 kinase inhibition, such as point mutations in the KD that impair drug binding or cellular/biological processes that interfere with TKI availability and result in suboptimal drug concentrations at the target. In contrast, BCR-ABL1–independent

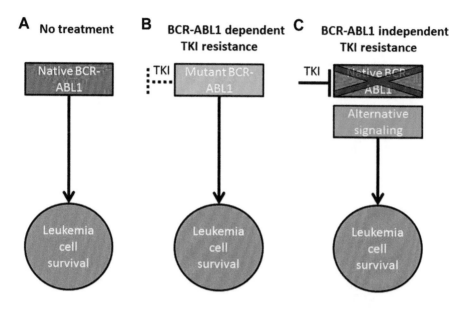

A No treatment **B** BCR-ABL1 dependent **C** BCR-ABL1 independent
TKI resistance   TKI resistance

Disease persistence

Fig. 1. BCR-ABL1–dependent versus BCR-ABL1–independent resistance. (*A*) Native BCR-ABL1 signaling in the absence of tyrosine kinase inhibitor (TKI) inhibition is necessary and suffi-cient for leukemogenesis in CML. (*B*) Kinase domain mutations in BCR-ABL1 can alter the binding of TKIs and lead to reconstitution of BCR-ABL1 signaling. (*C*) In the setting of effec-tive BCR-ABL1 inhibition with TKIs, leukemia cells persist owing to activation of alternative survival pathways.

resistance is mediated through alternative survival pathways operating in the context of effective TKI inhibition of BCR-ABL1. Overt clinical resistance is observed via both mechanisms, although acquired resistance is more likely to be BCR-ABL1 dependent, and primary resistance tends to be BCR-ABL1 independent. In BCR-ABL1–depen-dent resistance, achieving or restoring BCR-ABL1 inhibition is expected to induce or recapture responses, and the most effective approach is the use of alternate TKIs. For obvious reasons, this strategy in isolation will not be effective in BCR-ABL1–independent resistance. In this review, we discuss the mechanisms un-derlying BCR-ABL1–dependent and BCR-ABL1–independent resistance and the ther-apeutic strategies designed to circumvent them.

BCR-ABL1–Dependent Resistance

BCR-ABL1 kinase domain mutations
General considerations The active sites of tyrosine kinases exist in 2 principal confor-mations that are distinct by the position of key structural motifs, including the activa-tion loop (A-loop) that controls access of substrate to the catalytic site, the adenosine triphosphate (ATP)-binding loop (P-loop) and the highly conserved aspartate-phenylalanine-glycine (DFG) motif that coordinates an ATP-bound magnesium ion. In the inactive conformation, the activation loop is in a closed position, and the DFG in an outward ("DFG out") orientation. In contrast, in active kinases the A-loop is in an open conformation, and the DFG motif is oriented toward the catalytic site ("DFG-in") (**Fig. 2**).[9] Depending on whether they recognize an active or inactive kinase

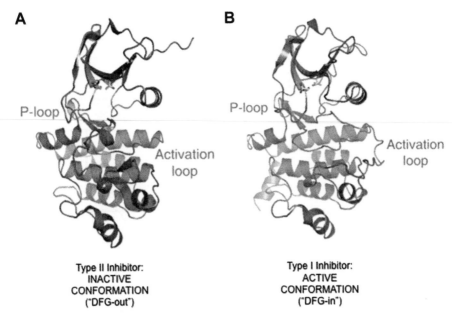

A

P-loop

Activation loop

Type II Inhibitor:
INACTIVE
CONFORMATION
("DFG-out")

B

P-loop

Activation loop

Type I Inhibitor:
ACTIVE
CONFORMATION
("DFG-in")

Fig. 2. Type I and type II inhibitors. (*A*) Type II inhibitors stabilize the inactive conformation of BCR-ABL1 in which the activation loop is closed and the aspartate-phenylalanine-glycine (DFG) is in an outward ("DFG out") orientation. (*B*) Type I inhibitors are ATP-competitive, binding to BCR-ABL1 when the activation loop is in an open position conformation and the DFG motif is oriented toward the catalytic site ("DFG-in"). (*Courtesy of* T. Clackson, PhD, Cambridge, MA.)

conformation, TKIs are referred to as type I or type II inhibitors, respectively.[10] Although all active site inhibitors are essentially ATP competitive, type II inhibitors could be considered as stabilizers of an inactive enzyme conformation, whereas type I inhibitors compete more directly with ATP for binding. Of the approved BCR-ABL1 TKIs, imatinib, nilotinib, and ponatinib are type II inhibitors, dasatinib is a type I inhibitor, and bosutinib exhibits features of both.[11–15] These general structural distinctions have practical consequences because they inform the number and types of mutations that confer resistance to a given TKI. Generally, type II inhibitors exhibit more stringent binding requirements, exposing more mutational vulnerabilities, but have the advantage of increased selectivity.[16] Type I inhibitors tend to be more promiscuous, but less prone to mutational escape.

Clinically observed BCR-ABL1 kinase domain mutations and structure–function relationships Anywhere from 50% to 90% of patients with CML who experience hematologic relapse on imatinib have been reported to harbor KD mutations.[17–20] Point substitutions at just 12 residues (M244, G250, Q252, Y253, E255, V299, F311, T315, F317, M351, F359, and H396) account for most resistance-associated KD mutations (**Fig. 3A**).[21] KD mutations develop with greater frequency in accelerated/blastic phase CML than in chronic phase CML.[18] For instance, a study of 297 patients with primary or acquired resistance to imatinib reported KD mutations in 27% of chronic phase patients, 52% of accelerated phase patients, 75% of myeloid blastic phase patients and 83% lymphoid blastic phase patients.[22] This suggests that reactivation of BCR-ABL1 signaling is critical to conferring an aggressive clinical phenotype. KD mutations can

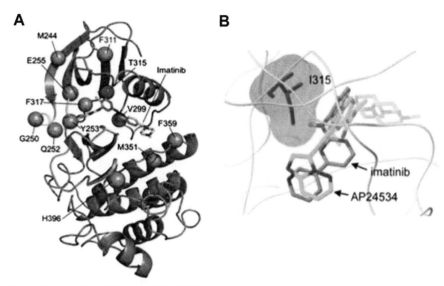

Fig. 3. Key residues influence BCR-ABL1–dependent resistance to tyrosine kinase inhibitors (TKIs). (*A*) Crystal structure of the ABL1 kinase domain in complex with imatinib. Twelve positions (in *orange*, T315 in *red*) account for most clinical BCR-ABL1 TKI resistance. The phosphate-binding (*yellow*) and activation loops (*green*) are indicated. (*B*) Superposition of imatinib and AP24534 (ponatinib) highlighting the effect of the Thr to Ile mutation. High-affinity binding of imatinib and other 2G TKIs to BCR-ABL1 requires a critical hydrogen bond with residue T315, which is eliminated upon the conversion of threonine to isoleucine. Unlike other clinically available TKIs, ponatinib does not form a hydrogen bond with T315 and has activity against the T315I mutant form of BCR-ABL1. (*From* [*A*] Zabriskie MS, Eide CA, Tantravahi SK, et al. BCR-ABL1 compound mutations combining key kinase domain positions confer clinical resistance to ponatinib in Ph chromosome-positive leukemia. Cancer Cell 2014;26(3):430, with permission; and [*B*] O'Hare T, Shakespeare WC, Zhu X, et al. AP24534, a pan-BCR-ABL inhibitor for chronic myeloid leukemia, potently inhibits the T315I mutant and overcomes mutation-based resistance. Cancer Cell 2009;16(5):403, with permission.)

also be detected at low levels in patients at diagnosis, and may in some cases become clinically relevant upon selection of clones by TKI therapy.[23,24] However, because this is not a predictable development, testing for KD mutations at diagnosis is not generally recommended.[5,24] Interestingly, the duration of disease before the initiation of TKI therapy correlates with the frequency of KD mutations, which supports a role for BCR-ABL1–induced self-mutagenesis.[18] Moreover, advanced phase CML, clonal cytogenetic evolution, and the KD mutation rate are correlated, suggesting a temporal relationship between uninhibited exposure to BCR-ABL1 kinase activity and degree of genomic instability.[25]

Of the approved TKIs, imatinib exhibits the broadest spectrum of vulnerabilities and more than 50 different imatinib-resistance KD mutations have been described.[26,27] Solving the crystal structure of ABL1 in complex with an imatinib analogue was critical for understanding KD mutation-based imatinib resistance. In contrast with expectations, imatinib was found to recognize an inactive kinase conformation, with the A-loop in a closed position. Additionally, there was extensive 'downward' displacement of the P-loop.[11] Last, imatinib was found to form a hydrogen bond with threonine 315. This binding mode is reflected in the types of KD mutations associated with imatinib resistance.[28] P-loop mutations are thought to prevent the structural adjustments required for optimal drug binding, the T315I mutant causes a steric clash and A-loop mutations stabilize the kinase in an active conformation from which imatinib is excluded. The degree of resistance conferred by the various KD mutations varies greatly, and some (such as M351 T or F311 L) remain amenable to dose escalation. In contrast, second-generation TKIs such as dasatinib and nilotinib retain inhibitory activity against the majority of mutants conferring imatinib resistance, with the notable exception of the T315I 'gatekeeper' mutation.[29] Nilotinib was developed from the imatinib scaffold, but has a much improved topological fit, greatly increasing binding affinity. As a result, nilotinib captures many imatinib resistant mutants, although their relative sensitivities to imatinib and nilotinib are similar.[13,30] Thus, nilotinib overcomes resistance through tighter binding to a very similar (inactive) ABL1 conformation. Dasatinib was initially reported to bind to ABL1 with less stringent conformational requirements compared with imatinib, but sophisticated nuclear MRI studies suggest it is a type I inhibitor.[12] The dasatinib resistance mutation spectrum is distinct and includes V299 and F317 as hotspots.[31] However, both nilotinib and dasatinib make a hydrogen bond with T315 and consequently have no activity against T315I. Bosutinib's resistance mutation spectrum is similar to that of dasatinib, suggesting that type I binding is dominant.[32] Ponatinib in contrast is a type II inhibitor that binds ABL1 in a conformation that is quite similar to that observed with imatinib, except that no hydrogen bond is formed with T315 (see **Fig. 3**B).[33] Owing to this and its high target affinity, ponatinib exhibits activity against all single BCR-ABL1 mutants at achievable plasma concentrations. In vitro mutagenesis assays developed by us and others fairly accurately predict clinical mutations, validating the fascinating link between structural analysis and clinical observations.[33] Clinically, the type of BCR-ABL1 mutation informs the selection of salvage therapy and represents a prime example of individualized cancer therapy. It is important to note, however, that the convenient heat maps displaying the differential activity of the approved TKIs toward the various KD mutants are a guide, but not a dogma (**Fig. 4**). For example, achievable plasma concentrations and plasma protein binding are additional variables not captured by in vitro assays of BCR-ABL1–expressing cell lines. Further, correlations are tight only toward the negative side. Thus, the presence of a T315I mutation predicts resistance, but there is no guarantee that a patient with a 'sensitive' mutant will respond to a given TKI. Failure to respond to TKI therapy in this setting could be owing to alternative BCR-ABL1–dependent mechanisms of resistance (eg, efflux pumps, see below), or to BCR-ABL1–independent mechanisms.

No single BCR-ABL1 KD mutation has been demonstrated to confer resistance to ponatinib. However, T315I-inclusive compound mutations, defined as a BCR-ABL1 allele with 2 or more mutations including T315I, have been associated with ponatinib failure[21] in advanced phase CML and Philadelphia chromosome-positive (PH+) acute lymphoblastic leukemia. A recent analysis of chronic phase patients with CML in the PACE trial failed to demonstrate that baseline compound mutation status, regardless of T315I inclusion, affects cytogenetic or molecular responses to ponatinib in this cohort.[34]

Increased BCR-ABL1 expression
Increased BCR-ABL1 expression via BCR-ABL1 gene amplification, Ph duplication, and differential regulation of oncogene transcription has been demonstrated in patients, but its relationship to acquired clinical resistance is less certain than in cases of KD mutations. High levels of the BCR-ABL1 oncoprotein are associated with more advanced phase disease, often preceding the development of overt resistance

IC50-fold increase (WT = 1)

		Imatinib	Bosutinib	Dasatinib	Nilotinib	Ponatinib
	Parental	10.8	38.3	568.3	38.4	570.0
	WT	1	1	1	1	1
P-loop	M244V	0.9	0.9	2.0	1.2	3.2
	L248R	14.6	22.9	12.5	30.2	6.2
	L248V	3.5	3.5	5.1	2.8	3.4
	G250E	6.9	4.3	4.4	4.6	6.0
	Q252H	1.4	0.8	3.1	2.6	6.1
	Y253F	3.6	1.0	1.6	3.2	3.7
	Y253H	8.7	0.6	2.6	36.9	2.6
	E255K	6.0	9.5	5.6	6.7	8.4
	E255V	17.0	5.5	3.4	10.3	12.9
C-helix	D276G	2.2	0.6	1.4	2.0	2.1
	E279K	3.6	1.0	1.6	2.0	3.0
	E292L	0.7	1.1	1.3	1.8	2.0
ATP binding region	V299L	1.5	26.1	8.7	1.3	0.6
	T315A	1.7	6.0	58.9	2.7	0.4
	T315I	17.5	45.4	75.0	39.4	3.0
	T315V	12.2	29.3	736.8	57.0	2.1
	F317L	2.6	2.4	4.5	2.2	0.7
	F317R	2.3	33.5	114.8	2.3	4.9
	F317V	0.4	11.5	21.3	0.5	2.3
SH2-contact	M343T	1.2	1.1	0.9	0.8	0.9
	M351T	1.8	0.7	0.9	0.4	1.2
Substrate binding region	F359I	6.0	2.9	3.0	16.3	2.9
	F359V	2.9	0.9	1.5	5.2	4.4
A-loop	L384M	1.3	0.5	2.2	2.3	2.2
	H396P	2.4	0.4	1.1	2.4	1.4
	H396R	3.9	0.8	1.6	3.1	5.9
C-terminal lobe	F486S	8.1	2.3	3.0	1.9	2.1
	L248R + F359I	11.7	39.3	13.7	96.2	17.7

Sensitive ≤2
Moderately resistant 2.1–4
Resistant 4.1–10
Highly resistant >10

via KD mutations.[35] Thus, higher levels of BCR-ABL1 may allow for sufficient kinase activity to persist despite the presence of TKIs, enabling leukemia cell survival until a KD mutation is acquired and confers overt resistance. One indication that these relationships are complex is the seemingly paradoxic observation that primary CD34+ CML cells engineered to express high levels of BCR-ABL1 have been reported to exhibit increased sensitivity to imatinib in vitro.[19,28,36,37]

Drug influx/efflux pumps

Organic-cation transporter-1 Organic-cation transporter-1 (OCT-1) is a cellular influx pump for imatinib that has been demonstrated to influence intracellular drug availability. Low OCT-1 activity imparts BCR-ABL1–dependent imatinib resistance. High OCT-1 activity is predictive of improved MMR rates, event-free survival, and overall survival in patients treated with imatinib.[38,39] Patients with low OCT-1 activity and imatinib trough plasma levels of less than 1200 ng/mL have inferior outcomes and benefit from imatinib dose intensification.[40] Imatinib trough levels of less than 1200 ng/mL do not necessarily predict inferior outcomes in patients with high OCT-1 activity and these patients are likely to meet molecular milestones on standard dose imatinib. OCT-1 does not regulate cellular uptake of dasatinib, nilotinib, or ponatinib.[41–43] In the future, baseline OCT-1 testing may identify candidates for trough imatinib monitoring and imatinib dose intensification, thereby avoiding unnecessary TKI switching owing to perceived imatinib failure, but it is not part of current routine clinical practice. Similarly, although several members of the ATP-binding cassette (ABC) transporter family, including ABCB1 and ABCG2, have been implicated in TKI resistance, testing for polymorphisms and increased expression of ABC transporters is not routine clinically.[27,37,43–50]

Tyrosine kinase inhibitor bioavailability All of the TKIs used in CML undergo extensive hepatic first-pass metabolism by CYP3A4 and strong inducers of CYP3A4 can contribute to TKI resistance. Patients on TKIs should undergo thorough medication reconciliation to avoid potential drug–drug interactions that can negatively impact TKI efficacy. Common CYP3A4-inducing medications and supplements include dexamethasone, rifampicin, phenobarbital, phenytoin, carbamazepine, and St. John's wort.[51] Gastric pH-modifying medications such as H2 antagonists and proton pump inhibitors can affect the bioavailability of dasatinib owing to the drug's poor solubility in solutions with a pH of greater than 4.0. These patients must be counseled to take antacids 2 hours before or 2 hours after dasatinib administration to avoid decreases in dasatinib exposure that can occur with their concomitant administration.[52,53]

BCR-ABL1–Independent Resistance

General considerations

Point mutations in BCR-ABL1 are an important mechanism of TKI resistance in CML, but nearly 40% of cases of clinical TKI failure occur in the setting of sustained

---

Fig. 4. Activity of tyrosine kinase inhibitors (TKIs) against mutant isoforms of BCR-ABL1 in Ba/F3 cells. The relative increase in median inhibition concentration (IC50) value over wild-type (WT) BCR-ABL1 is depicted for each TKI against single BCR-ABL1 mutants. Green indicates sensitive mutants, yellow indicates moderate resistance, orange indicates resistance, and red indicates marked resistance. In patients, TKI efficacy depends on other factors, such as oral and cellular bioavailability. (*From* Eiring AM, Deininger MW. Individualizing kinase-targeted cancer therapy: the paradigm of chronic myeloid leukemia. Genome Biol 2014;15(9):461; with permission.)

BCR-ABL1 inhibition.[54] In this scenario, activation of alternative survival pathways must be responsible for primary or secondary resistance. Conceptually, CML cell survival can be mediated through cell-autonomous (leukemia cell intrinsic) mechanisms or through cell-extrinsic microenvironmental factors provided by the bone marrow niche.[55] It is worth noting that although BCR-ABL1 independent resistance can confer overt resistance in active disease, it is also an important contributor to MRD, likely accounting for leukemia stem cell (LSC) persistence despite DMR to TKI therapy. Multiple (and counting) signaling pathways have been implicated in BCR-ABL1–independent resistance (**Table 1**). We have proposed that various upstream pathways may converge on common downstream mediators, offering therapeutic opportunities despite the diversity of upstream signaling.[56] Moreover, it seems that the pathways activated by extrinsic and intrinsic resistance mechanisms overlap. In this frame of thinking, extrinsic resistance may enable the survival of leukemogenic cells despite TKI inhibition of BCR-ABL1, until the surviving cells manage to activate the very same pathway through cell-intrinsic mechanisms, leading to overt resistance.

STAT3

STAT3 activation has been demonstrated to impart survival cues to leukemic cells via cell-intrinsic and extrinsic mechanisms. Coculture of TKI-sensitive CML primary cells with HS-5 human bone marrow stromal cells was shown to promote $STAT3^{Y705}$ phosphorylation and leukemia cell survival through soluble bone marrow–derived factors despite BCR-ABL1 inhibition.[57,58] Moreover, in the absence of bone marrow–derived factors, BCR-ABL1–independent activation of STAT3 was demonstrated to be a recurring feature of TKI-resistant cell lines and primary CML cells from patients with clinical resistance to multiple TKIs, suggesting that cell-autonomous activation of STAT3 can mediate CML cell survival.[56] Thus, consistent with the concepts described above, prosurvival cues seem to converge on STAT3 as a crucial distal signal integrator and arbiter of drug resistance. As a result, synthetic lethality approaches designed to inhibit both BCR-ABL1 and $pSTAT3^{Y705}$ hold therapeutic potential, both in active disease and as a tactic to eliminate MRD.

PI3K/AKT

PI3K signaling is required for the proliferation and growth of CML cells.[59] Activation of the PI3K/AKT/mammalian target of rapamycin pathway has been shown to facilitate primary CML cell survival during imatinib treatment until overt resistance through secondary mutations emerges.[60] Cotreatment of CML primary cells with nilotinib and the PI3K inhibitor NVP-BEZ235 was shown to inhibit cell growth and increase apoptosis.[61] Increased cytoplasmic retention of FOXO1, a transcription factor downstream of the PI3K signaling axis, has been reported to contribute to BCR-ABL1–independent resistance in TKI-resistant CML cell lines.[54] Elevation in FOXO1 levels has also been demonstrated in primary cells from relapsed patients with CML lacking BCR-ABL1 KD mutations. TKI-resistant cells seem to be sensitive to combination drug strategies involving BCR-ABL1 TKIs and PI3K inhibitors that facilitate nuclear translocation of FOXO1.

RAF/MEK/ERK

Enhanced MAP kinase signaling has previously been observed in imatinib-treated CD34+ CML progenitor cells.[62] More recently, Ma and colleagues[63] performed a large-scale RNA interference screen that revealed increased RAF/MEK/ERK pathway activity mediated through PRKCH in BCR-ABL1–independent imatinib-resistant CML cell lines and patient samples. They found that dual treatment with imatinib and the MEK inhibitor trametinib preferentially killed human CML CD34+ cells while sparing

Table 1
Targets for eradication of LSCs in CML

Target	References	Trial	Drug(s) Tested	Comments
Wnt/β-catenin	Zhao et al,[72] 2007; Lim et al,[73] 2013	+	PRI-724	Difficult target
MNK				
Hedgehog	Dierks et al,[84] 2008; Zhao et al,[72] 2009 Nature	+	BMS-833923 LDE225	Failed (toxicity)
5-Lipoxygenase	Chen et al,[85] 2009	+	Zileuton	Currently recruiting
BCL6	Hurtz et al,[96] 2011 JExMed	—	RI-BPI	Small molecule inhibitor in development
MYC	Reavie et al,[94] 2013; Abraham et al,[95] 2016	—	—	Difficult target
PP2A	Neviani et al,[86] 2013; Neviani et al,[97] 2007 J Clin Invest	—	—	Fingolimod approved for MS
PPAR-γ	Prost et al,[2015][128]	+	Pioglitazone	Ongoing
SIRT1	Li et al,[89] 2012 Cancer Cell	+	Panobinostat Vorinostat	Tested in refractory CML
Rad52	Cramer-Morales et al,[87] 2013	—	—	—
MEK	Ma et al,[63] 2014; Packer et al,[64] 2011	+	MEK-162	Ongoing
BCL2 family	Goff et al,[98] 2013 Cancer Stem Cell	+	Obatoclax	Tested in advanced hematologic malignancies, including CML-BC
Autophagy	Bellodi et al,[90] 2009	+	Hydroxychloroquine	Ongoing (CHOICES)
PML	Ito et al,[91] 2008	+	As$_2$O$_3$	Ongoing
JAK2	Traer et al,[57] 2012; Neviani et al,[86] 2013	+	Ruxolitinib	Ongoing
ADAR1	Jiang et al,[93] 2013	—	—	—
STAT3	Eiring et al,[56] 2014	—	—	Difficult target
EZH2	Xie et al,[69] 2016; Scott et al,[68] 2016	—	—	—
Heat shock proteins	Peng et al,[88] 2007	+	STA-9090	Ongoing
Fap1	Huang et al,[92] 2016	—	—	—
BCR-ABL1	Pinilla-Ibarz et al,[118] 2000; Bocchia et al,[119] 2005	+	Breakpoint peptide vaccines	Suggestion of activity

				Negative studies
PR1	Molldrem et al,[120] 2000; Rezvani et al,[121] 2011	+	Peptide vaccines	
WT1	Gao et al,[122] 2000; Dubrovsky et al,[123] 2014	+	Peptide vaccines Peptide-specific antibody WT transduced autologous T cells	Ongoing (some)
IL1RAP	Järås M et al,[124] 2010	—	Antibody	—
IL3R (CD123)	Frolova et al,[125] 2014	—	DT-conjugated antibody (SL-401; SL-501)	—

Abbreviations: CML, chronic myeloid leukemia; LSC, leukemic stem cell; MS, multiple sclerosis; PPAR-γ, peroxisome proliferator-activated receptor-γ; WT, wild type.

normal hematopoietic cells and prolonged survival in their murine models of BCR-ABL1–independent imatinib-resistant CML. In line with this, another study described paradoxic RAS-dependent activation of the RAF/MEK/ERK pathway in nilotinib-treated primary CML cells containing T315I and found that nilotinib synergizes with MEK inhibition to induce synthetic lethality in these cells.[64] In TKI-sensitive CML cells, MEK activity seems to facilitate BCR-ABL1–mediated oncogene addiction, suggesting that activation of this pathway is critical for leukemia cell survival and a potential target for combination drug inhibition strategies.[65]

Nucleocytoplasmic transport

More recently, *XPO1* and *RAN*, components of the nucleocytoplasmic transport complex, were identified as genes whose shRNA-mediated knockdown decreased cell proliferation in a BCR-ABL1–independent imatinib-resistant cell line.[66] Both shRNA-mediated inhibition of RAN and treatment with the XPO1 inhibitor KPT-330 (selinexor) increased the sensitivity of resistant cells to imatinib. KPT-330 has also demonstrated preclinical antileukemic activity in mouse models of CML and was observed to decrease leukocytosis and palliate symptoms in a TKI-resistant patient with accelerated phase CML who was provided the drug on a compassionate use basis.[67]

EZH2

EZH2, a histone methyltransferase that provides the catalytic subunit of polycomb repressive complex 2, has been shown to be overexpressed in CML LSCs. Two recent publications have highlighted the importance of EZH2 misregulation and its association with reprogramming of H3K27me3 targets in LSCs, resulting in LSC protection from apoptosis and TKI resistance.[68,69] EZH2 inactivation was shown to delay the development of leukemia and prolong survival in mouse models of CML independent of BCR-ABL1 mutational status. In mice with preexisting gene inactivation of *EZH2* through CRISPR/Cas9-mediated gene editing there was slowed disease progression and extended survival. Combination treatment with nilotinib and EZH2 inhibitors in CML primary cells engrafted into NOD/SCID mice led to a greater reduction of the LSC population compared with nilotinib treatment alone. Normal hematopoietic stem and progenitor cells seem to be spared from EZH2 inhibition, perhaps owing to compensation from EZH1, which is expressed at higher levels in normal HSCs compared with LSCs. The selective vulnerability of LSCs to EZH2 inhibition may provide a therapeutic window to eradicate TKI-persistent LSCs with minimal effects on normal hematopoiesis.

Numerous other BCR-ABL1 independent factors have been proposed to contribute to CML LSC persistence and TKI resistance, including activation of SRC family kinases, Wnt–β-catenin, hypoxia-inducible factor 1α, arachidonate 15-lipoxygenase, miR-126, p53, MYC, ADAR1, SIRT1, RAD21 heat shock proteins, PP2A, Fap1, apoptotic regulators, the Hedgehog pathway, and the IL-2/CD25 signaling circuit.[55,70–95] The number of theoretic synthetic lethality approaches involving TKIs and other inhibitors is destined to increase as new resistance mechanisms are unearthed, yet it remains unclear which combinations harbor clinical potential above and beyond TKI monotherapy.

New Therapies

Tyrosine kinase inhibitors

ABL001 One of the most anticipated new therapies for CML is ABL001, a novel allosteric inhibitor of BCR-ABL1 targeting the myristoyl pocket of the ABL1 kinase. In physiologic conditions, the myristoylated *N*-terminus of ABL1 serves to negatively regulate kinase activity, but is lost upon fusion with BCR in CML. ABL001 was designed to restore this autoregulatory function to the BCR-ABL1 fusion protein, thereby inhibiting oncogenic signaling. Single-agent ABL001 led to tumor regression in mice xenografted with the KCL22 CML cell line, although all tumors eventually recurred. The in vivo combination treatment with nilotinib and ABL001 induced complete and sustained regression of disease in mice, with no relapses observed as long as 5 months out from active drug treament.[99] These encouraging results led to a dose-finding phase I trial of ABL001 monotherapy in chronic phase and accelerated phase patients with CML with failure of 2 or more TKIs owing to resistance or intolerance.[100] More than 50% of patients enrolled had failed 3 or more TKIs. Initial results from the trial are promising: 82% of TKI-resistant patients in cytogenetic relapse achieved MCyR by 3 months, including 55% who achieved CCyR. Nearly 30% of TKI-resistant patients achieved MMR by 5 months, and clinical activity was pronounced across a range of mutations. A single relapse was attributed to a mutation in the myristoyl pocket.[100] Overall, the drug was well-tolerated, with common grade 3 toxicities, including lipase elevation and cytopenias. At the time of last reporting, the maximum tolerated dose had not been reached. Other arms of the phase I study are assessing the safety and tolerability of ABL001 in combination with imatinib, nilotinib, and dasatinib.

Several other TKIs were previously in development for CML, including bafetinib (BCR-ABL1/Lyn inhibitor) and rebastinib (ABL1/TIE2 inhibitor), but have been side-lined owing to poor efficacy in early phase clinical trials.[101,102] A phase I trial of the intravenous ABL1/Aurora kinase inhibitor danusertib produced modest responses in T315I-positive, TKI-resistant accelerated phase/BC CML and Ph+ acute lymphoblastic leukemia.[103] The vascular endothelial growth factor receptor inhibitor axitinib has been found to inhibit BCR-ABL1 mutants with substitutions at positions 315 and 299, but its clinical use is limited by this mutational selectivity.[104,105] Radotinib, a second-generation oral BCR-ABL1 inhibitor with an almost identical chemical structure as nilotinib, is approved for second-line treatment of CML in South Korea. An ongoing phase III study investigating radotinib versus imatinib in newly diagnosed CML demonstrated superior 12-month CCyR and MMR rates with radotinib 300 mg 2 times a day (CCyR, 91% vs 76%; MMR, 52% vs 30%).[106] Not surprisingly, the in vitro efficacy of radotinib against single BCR-ABL1 mutants seems to be similar to that of nilotinib.[107]

Drug combinations to eradicate leukemic stem cells and eliminate minimal residual disease

Patients who have maintained long-term (1–2 years minimum) DMR on TKI therapy may be candidates for TKI discontinuation. When treated with single-agent TKI therapy, at best one-half of newly diagnosed patients with CML will eventually be eligible for TKI discontinuation trials, and of these, at most 50% to 60% will successfully maintain treatment-free remission (TFR) at 1 year after TKI discontinuation.[108] The finding that a portion of patients are "operationally cured" after TKI treatment is surprising given the wealth of data suggesting CML LSCs are not eradicated by BCR-ABL1 inhibition. It also remains unclear why patients with seemingly identical deep responses segregate in their responses to TKI discontinuation. Recent data have emerged to support the role of immune surveillance by natural killer and T cells in maintaining successful TFR, implying that alternative biological factors contribute to optimal disease control.[109] Various TKI discontinuation trials are ongoing, and attempts to clarify the clinical and biologic characteristics predictive of successful TFR are reflected in a trend toward more liberalized patient eligibility criteria and an emphasis on correlative studies (**Table 2**).

Table 2
Summary of TKI discontinuation studies

Trial	Patients Reported	Treatment Before Discontinuation	Eligibility for TKI Discontinuation by MR	Threshold for Restarting TKI	TFR% (Median Follow-up Time)
Imatinib discontinuation trials					
STIM1	100	Imatinib ± prior IFN	MR^5 (≥ 2 y)	≥ 2 consecutive samples with detectable PCR and a 1-log increase	39% (55 mo)
STIM2	124	Imatinib	$MR^{4.5}$ (≥ 2 y)	≥ 2 consecutive samples with detectable PCR and a 1-log increase	46% (2 y)
TWISTER	40	Imatinib ± prior IFN	$MR^{4.5}$ (≥ 2 y)	Detectable PCR	45% (42 mo)
A-STIM	80	Imatinib ± prior IFN	Undetectable PCR (≥ 2 y) with low level positives occasionally allowed	Loss of MMR	64% (23 mo)
ISAV	112	Imatinib	Undetectable PCR (18 mo)	Loss of MMR	51.9% at 36 mo (21 mo)
KID	90	Imatinib ± prior IFN	$MR^{4.5}$ (≥ 2 y)	Loss of MMR	50% (26.6 mo)
HOVON	18	Imatinib	$MR^{4.5}$ (≥ 2 y)	Detectable PCR	33% (36 mo)
Imatinib and/or 2G-TKI discontinuation trials					
STOP-2G TKI	52	Nilotinib or dasatinib	$MR^{4.5}$ (≥ 2 y)	Loss of MMR	61% (6 mo); ongoing
ENEST Freedom	190	Nilotinib	$MR^{4.5}$ (≥ 1 y)	Loss of MMR	51.6% (week 48); ongoing
ENESTop	126	Second-line nilotinib	$MR^{4.5}$ (≥ 1 y)	Loss of MMR or confirmed loss of MR^4	57.9% (week 48); ongoing
ENEST Path	1058 (estimated)	Imatinib followed by nilotinib	MR^4 (≥ 1-2 y)	Loss of MMR or confirmed loss of MR^4	Ongoing
ENEST Goal	300 (estimated)	Imatinib without MMR followed by nilotinib	$MR^{4.5}$ (≥ 1-2 y)	Confirmed loss of MR^4	Ongoing
DADI	63	Second-line dasatinib	MR^4 (≥ 1 y)	Loss of MR^4	49% (6 mo)
DASFREE	79 (estimated)	Dasatinib	$MR^{4.5}$ (≥ 1 y)	Loss of MMR	Ongoing

CMLV (TIGER)	652 (estimated)	Nilotinib vs nilotinib + IFN	MR^4 (≥ 1 y)	Loss of MMR	Ongoing
LAST	173 (estimated)	Imatinib, nilotinib, dasatinib or bosutinib	MR^4 (≥ 2 y)	Detectable PCR	Ongoing
DESTINY	168 (estimated)	Imatinib. nilotinib or dasatinib	Patients in MMR or MR^4 (≥ 1 y) who can maintain MMR response on half-dose TKI for 12 mo	Loss of MMR	Ongoing
EURO-SKI	200	Imatinib, nilotinib or dasatinib	MR^4 (≥ 1 y)	Loss of MMR	61% (6 mo); ongoing

Abbreviations: IFN, interferon; MMR, major molecular response; MR, molecular response; PCR, polymerase chain reaction; TFR, treatment-free remission; TKI, tyrosine kinase inhibitor.

Adapted from Saußele S, Richter J, Hochhaus A, et al. The concept of treatment-free remission in chronic myeloid leukemia. Leukemia 2016;30(8):1641; with permission.

TKI discontinuation is an evolving goal of CML therapy and has been embraced by patients motivated to come off these chronic medications owing to undesirable side effects, which, in some cases, can be quite serious (ie, pulmonary hypertension on dasatinib or arterial occlusive events on nilotinib). The reality that the majority of patients with CML will never attain TFR with current therapies has led to efforts to combine TKIs with other drugs in hopes of eliminating TKI-persistent LSCs and the reservoir of cells responsible for MRD.

Tyrosine kinase inhibitors plus immune therapies Before imatinib, interferon-α (IFN) based therapy was standard of care for CML. Anecdotal evidence suggests that IFN preferentially targets leukemic stem cells in CML, as demonstrated by the fact a small minority of patients with CML treated with IFN alone were functionally cured of their disease.[110] Randomized trials of imatinib and pegylated IFN report improved molecular response rates with combination therapy compared with imatinib alone.[111,112] With the advent of TKI discontinuation and documentation of successful TFRs, there has been renewed interest in pegylated IFN as an adjunct to TKI therapy in promoting DMR. This had led to early phase trials investigating pegylated IFN in combination with second-generation TKIs. Nonrandomized trials of nilotinib or dasatinib in combination with pegylated IFN in newly diagnosed patients with CML have reported 12-month MR$^{4.5}$ rates of 17% and 27% to 30%, respectively, which compare favorably to the 12-month MR$^{4.5}$ rates observed in the registration trials of frontline nilotinib (ENESTnd) and dasatinib (DASISION).[113–117] A phase III randomized trial of IFN in combination with nilotinib is underway in Germany. There remains considerable interest in developing novel immune therapies against a variety of tumor antigens and while early phase trials investigating peptide vaccines have had mixed results, antibody-based treatments may hold promise.[118–125]

Tyrosine kinase inhibitors plus inhibitors of additional pathways Despite mounting evidence implicating diverse pathways in BCR-ABL1–independent resistance and LSC persistence, there are a limited number of clinical trials investigating inhibitors of these pathways in combination with TKIs.

Leukemic stem and progenitor cells may be protected in the bone marrow niche via JAK2/STAT5 activation by exogenous growth factors in the setting of BCR-ABL1 inhibition.[57,126,127] CML CD34$^+$ cells display reduced engraftment when treated ex vivo with the combination of TKI and ruxolitinib (a clinically available JAK2 inhibitor) and transplanted into NSG mice.[127] The impact of the addition of ruxolitinib to baseline TKI therapy in CML is being studied in a phase 1/2 trial (NCT01751425) and the specific combination of ruxolitinib and nilotinib in CML and Ph$^+$ acute lymphoblastic leukemia is being investigated in a separate phase I/II study (NCT02253277).

Pioglitazone, an agonist of peroxisome proliferator-activated receptor-γ belonging to the glitazone family of antidiabetic drugs, has been found to induce apoptosis in LSCs when used in combination with imatinib, presumably by downregulating STAT5 transcriptional targets, including HIF2α and CITED2.[128] The addition of pioglitazone to TKI therapy in 3 patients with CML unable to reach CMR after several years of continuous imatinib treatment was associated with sustained MR$^{4.5}$ in all 3 patients at 6 months to 1 year after initial pioglitazone exposure. These findings led to a phase II trial combining imatinib and pioglitazone in patients with persistent MRD on imatinib. The incidence of polymerase chain reaction negativity was reported at 57% for the combination group and 27% for a historical cohort receiving imatinib alone. Currently there are several trials investigating pioglitazone in combination with TKIs for CML, including 1 study (PIO2STOP) attempting to define its use in a second trial of TKI discontinuation for patients who experienced loss of MMR after initial TKI discontinuation.

SUMMARY

Owing to improved survival, the prevalence of CML is estimated to exceed 180,000 cases by 2050, thereby establishing CML as the most common form of leukemia in the United States.[129] Although excellent progress has been made through the introduction of targeted molecular therapy over the last 2 decades, new strategies to eliminate MRD and increase the pool of candidates eligible for trials of TFR are needed. Eliminating TKI resistance and LSC persistence by dual targeting of BCR-ABL1 and alternative pathways seems to be the most promising therapeutic avenue to decrease leukemic disease burden and potentiate "operational cures." The number of alternative pathways posited to establish synthetic lethality with TKIs is overwhelming, and it will take time and effort to sift through the multiple permutations with rigorous clinical testing. Ultimately, though, responses to cancer therapy depend not just on the efficacy of target inhibition, but also on factors such as patient compliance and tolerability of side effects that need to be addressed with a completely different set of tools. It is for these reasons that mechanisms of resistance will always keep pace with therapeutic developments, and we will be contending with them for as long as we continue our fight against cancer.

REFERENCES

1. SEER cancer statistics factsheets: chronic myeloid leukemia. Bethesda (MD): National Cancer Institute. Available at: http://seer.cancer.gov/statfacts/html/cmyl.html. Accessed November 17, 2016.
2. Ren R. Mechanisms of BCR-ABL in the pathogenesis of chronic myelogenous leukaemia. Nat Rev Cancer 2005;5:172–83.
3. Bower H, Bjorkholm M, Dickman PW, et al. Life expectancy of patients with chronic myeloid leukemia approaches the life expectancy of the general population. J Clin Oncol 2016;34:2851–7.
4. Steegmann JL, Baccarani M, Breccia M, et al. European LeukemiaNet recommendations for the management and avoidance of adverse events of treatment in chronic myeloid leukaemia. Leukemia 2016;30(8):1648–71.
5. Baccarani M, Deininger MW, Rosti G, et al. European LeukemiaNet recommendations for the management of chronic myeloid leukemia: 2013. Blood 2013;122:872–84.
6. O'Brien S, Radich JP, Abboud CN, et al. Chronic myelogenous leukemia, version 1.2015. J Natl Compr Canc Netw 2014;12:1590–610.
7. Press RD, Galderisi C, Yang R, et al. A half-log increase in BCR-ABL RNA predicts a higher risk of relapse in patients with chronic myeloid leukemia with an imatinib-induced complete cytogenetic response. Clin Cancer Res 2007;13:6136–43.
8. Hochhaus A. Chronic myelogenous leukemia (CML): resistance to tyrosine kinase inhibitors. Ann Oncol 2006;17(Suppl 10):x274–9.
9. Treiber DK, Shah NP. Ins and outs of kinase DFG motifs. Chem Biol 2013;20:745–6.
10. Zhang J, Yang PL, Gray NS. Targeting cancer with small molecule kinase inhibitors. Nat Rev Cancer 2009;9:28–39.
11. Schindler T, Bornmann W, Pellicena P, et al. Structural mechanism for STI-571 inhibition of abelson tyrosine kinase. Science 2000;289:1938–42.
12. Vajpai N, Strauss A, Fendrich G, et al. Solution conformations and dynamics of ABL kinase-inhibitor complexes determined by NMR substantiate the different

binding modes of imatinib/nilotinib and dasatinib. J Biol Chem 2008;283: 18292–302.

13. Weisberg E, Manley PW, Breitenstein W, et al. Characterization of AMN107, a selective inhibitor of native and mutant Bcr-Abl. Cancer Cell 2005;7:129–41.

14. Levinson NM, Boxer SG. Structural and spectroscopic analysis of the kinase inhibitor bosutinib and an isomer of bosutinib binding to the Abl tyrosine kinase domain. PLoS One 2012;7:e29828.

15. Zhou T, Commodore L, Huang WS, et al. Structural mechanism of the Pan-BCR-ABL inhibitor ponatinib (AP24534): lessons for overcoming kinase inhibitor resistance. Chem Biol Drug Des 2011;77:1–11.

16. Davis MI, Hunt JP, Herrgard S, et al. Comprehensive analysis of kinase inhibitor selectivity. Nat Biotechnol 2011;29:1046–51.

17. Shah NP, Nicoll JM, Nagar B, et al. Multiple BCR-ABL kinase domain mutations confer polyclonal resistance to the tyrosine kinase inhibitor imatinib (STI571) in chronic phase and blast crisis chronic myeloid leukemia. Cancer Cell 2002;2: 117–25.

18. Branford S, Rudzki Z, Walsh S, et al. Detection of BCR-ABL mutations in patients with CML treated with imatinib is virtually always accompanied by clinical resistance, and mutations in the ATP phosphate-binding loop (P-loop) are associated with a poor prognosis. Blood 2003;102:276–83.

19. Hochhaus A, Kreil S, Corbin AS, et al. Molecular and chromosomal mechanisms of resistance to imatinib (STI571) therapy. Leukemia 2002;16:2190–6.

20. von Bubnoff N, Peschel C, Duyster J. Resistance of Philadelphia-chromosome positive leukemia towards the kinase inhibitor imatinib (STI571, Glivec): a targeted oncoprotein strikes back. Leukemia 2003;17:829–38.

21. Zabriskie MS, Eide CA, Tantravahi SK, et al. BCR-ABL1 compound mutations combining key kinase domain positions confer clinical resistance to ponatinib in Ph chromosome-positive leukemia. Cancer Cell 2014;26:428–42.

22. Soverini S, Colarossi S, Gnani A, et al. Contribution of ABL kinase domain mutations to imatinib resistance in different subsets of Philadelphia-positive patients: by the GIMEMA Working Party on Chronic Myeloid Leukemia. Clin Cancer Res 2006;12:7374–9.

23. Roche-Lestienne C, Soenen-Cornu V, Grardel-Duflos N, et al. Several types of mutations of the Abl gene can be found in chronic myeloid leukemia patients resistant to STI571, and they can pre-exist to the onset of treatment. Blood 2002;100:1014–8.

24. Willis SG, Lange T, Demehri S, et al. High-sensitivity detection of BCR-ABL kinase domain mutations in imatinib-naive patients: correlation with clonal cytogenetic evolution but not response to therapy. Blood 2005;106:2128–37.

25. O'Hare T, Eide CA, Deininger MW. Bcr-Abl kinase domain mutations, drug resistance, and the road to a cure for chronic myeloid leukemia. Blood 2007;110: 2242–9.

26. O'Hare T, Zabriskie MS, Eiring AM, et al. Pushing the limits of targeted therapy in chronic myeloid leukaemia. Nat Rev Cancer 2012;12:513–26.

27. Apperley JF. Part I: mechanisms of resistance to imatinib in chronic myeloid leukaemia. Lancet Oncol 2007;8:1018–29.

28. Gorre ME, Mohammed M, Ellwood K, et al. Clinical resistance to STI-571 cancer therapy caused by BCR-ABL gene mutation or amplification. Science 2001;293: 876–80.

29. Eide CA, O'Hare T. Chronic myeloid leukemia: advances in understanding disease biology and mechanisms of resistance to tyrosine kinase inhibitors. Curr Hematol Malig Rep 2015;10:158–66.

30. Weisberg E, Manley P, Mestan J, et al. AMN107 (nilotinib): a novel and selective inhibitor of BCR-ABL. Br J Cancer 2006;94:1765–9.

31. Jabbour E, Hochhaus A, Cortes J, et al. Choosing the best treatment strategy for chronic myeloid leukemia patients resistant to imatinib: weighing the efficacy and safety of individual drugs with BCR-ABL mutations and patient history. Leukemia 2010;24:6–12.

32. Redaelli S, Piazza R, Rostagno R, et al. Activity of bosutinib, dasatinib, and nilotinib against 18 imatinib-resistant BCR/ABL mutants. J Clin Oncol 2009;27: 469–71.

33. O'Hare T, Shakespeare WC, Zhu X, et al. AP24534, a pan-BCR-ABL inhibitor for chronic myeloid leukemia, potently inhibits the T315I mutant and overcomes mutation-based resistance. Cancer Cell 2009;16:401–12.

34. Deininger MW, Hodgson JG, Shah NP, et al. Compound mutations in BCR-ABL1 are not major drivers of primary or secondary resistance to ponatinib in CP-CML patients. Blood 2016;127:703–12.

35. Barnes DJ, Palaiologou D, Panousopoulou E, et al. Bcr-Abl expression levels determine the rate of development of resistance to imatinib mesylate in chronic myeloid leukemia. Cancer Res 2005;65:8912–9.

36. Modi H, McDonald T, Chu S, et al. Role of BCR/ABL gene-expression levels in determining the phenotype and imatinib sensitivity of transformed human hematopoietic cells. Blood 2007;109:5411–21.

37. Milojkovic D, Apperley J. Mechanisms of resistance to imatinib and second-generation tyrosine inhibitors in chronic myeloid leukemia. Clin Cancer Res 2009;15:7519–27.

38. White DL, Dang P, Engler J, et al. Functional activity of the OCT-1 protein is predictive of long-term outcome in patients with chronic-phase chronic myeloid leukemia treated with imatinib. J Clin Oncol 2010;28:2761–7.

39. White DL, Saunders VA, Dang P, et al. Most CML patients who have a suboptimal response to imatinib have low OCT-1 activity: higher doses of imatinib may overcome the negative impact of low OCT-1 activity. Blood 2007;110:4064–72.

40. White DL, Radich J, Soverini S, et al. Chronic phase chronic myeloid leukemia patients with low OCT-1 activity randomized to high-dose imatinib achieve better responses and have lower failure rates than those randomized to standard-dose imatinib. Haematologica 2012;97:907–14.

41. White DL, Saunders VA, Dang P, et al. OCT-1-mediated influx is a key determinant of the intracellular uptake of imatinib but not nilotinib (AMN107): reduced OCT-1 activity is the cause of low in vitro sensitivity to imatinib. Blood 2006; 108:697–704.

42. Hiwase DK, Saunders V, Hewett D, et al. Dasatinib cellular uptake and efflux in chronic myeloid leukemia cells: therapeutic implications. Clin Cancer Res 2008; 14:3881–8.

43. Lu L, Saunders VA, Leclercq TM, et al. Ponatinib is not transported by ABCB1, ABCG2 or OCT-1 in CML cells. Leukemia 2015;29:1792–4.

44. Eadie LN, Hughes TP, White DL. Interaction of the efflux transporters ABCB1 and ABCG2 with imatinib, nilotinib, and dasatinib. Clin Pharmacol Ther 2014; 95:294–306.

45. Sen R, Natarajan K, Bhullar J, et al. The novel BCR-ABL and FLT3 inhibitor ponatinib is a potent inhibitor of the MDR-associated ATP-binding cassette transporter ABCG2. Mol Cancer Ther 2012;11:2033–44.

46. Eadie LN, Dang P, Saunders VA, et al. The clinical significance of ABCB1 overexpression in predicting outcome of CML patients undergoing first-line imatinib treatment. Leukemia 2017;31(1):75–82.

47. Giannoudis A, Davies A, Harris RJ, et al. The clinical significance of ABCC3 as an imatinib transporter in chronic myeloid leukaemia. Leukemia 2014;28: 1360–3.

48. Agrawal M, Hanfstein B, Erben P, et al. MDR1 expression predicts outcome of Ph+ chronic phase CML patients on second-line nilotinib therapy after imatinib failure. Leukemia 2014;28:1478–85.

49. Ni LN, Li JY, Miao KR, et al. Multidrug resistance gene (MDR1) polymorphisms correlate with imatinib response in chronic myeloid leukemia. Med Oncol 2011; 28:265–9.

50. Dulucq S, Bouchet S, Turcq B, et al. Multidrug resistance gene (MDR1) polymorphisms are associated with major molecular responses to standard-dose imatinib in chronic myeloid leukemia. Blood 2008;112:2024–7.

51. Haouala A, Widmer N, Duchosal MA, et al. Drug interactions with the tyrosine kinase inhibitors imatinib, dasatinib, and nilotinib. Blood 2011;117:e75–87.

52. Takahashi N, Miura M, Niioka T, et al. Influence of H2-receptor antagonists and proton pump inhibitors on dasatinib pharmacokinetics in Japanese leukemia patients. Cancer Chemother Pharmacol 2012;69:999–1004.

53. Eley T, Luo FR, Agrawal S, et al. Phase I study of the effect of gastric acid pH modulators on the bioavailability of oral dasatinib in healthy subjects. J Clin Pharmacol 2009;49:700–9.

54. Wagle M, Eiring AM, Wongchenko M, et al. A role for FOXO1 in BCR-ABL1-independent tyrosine kinase inhibitor resistance in chronic myeloid leukemia. Leukemia 2016;30:1493–501.

55. Eiring AM, Khorashad JS, Anderson DJ, et al. Beta-Catenin is required for intrinsic but not extrinsic BCR-ABL1 kinase-independent resistance to tyrosine kinase inhibitors in chronic myeloid leukemia. Leukemia 2015;29:2328–37.

56. Eiring AM, Kraft IL, Page BD, et al. STAT3 as a mediator of BCR-ABL1-independent resistance in chronic myeloid leukemia. Leuk Suppl 2014; 3:S5–6.

57. Traer E, MacKenzie R, Snead J, et al. Blockade of JAK2-mediated extrinsic survival signals restores sensitivity of CML cells to ABL inhibitors. Leukemia 2012; 26:1140–3.

58. Bewry NN, Nair RR, Emmons MF, et al. Stat3 contributes to resistance toward BCR-ABL inhibitors in a bone marrow microenvironment model of drug resistance. Mol Cancer Ther 2008;7:3169–75.

59. Skorski T, Kanakaraj P, Nieborowska-Skorska M, et al. Phosphatidylinositol-3 kinase activity is regulated by BCR/ABL and is required for the growth of Philadelphia chromosome-positive cells. Blood 1995;86:726–36.

60. Burchert A, Wang Y, Cai D, et al. Compensatory PI3-kinase/Akt/mTor activation regulates imatinib resistance development. Leukemia 2005;19:1774–82.

61. Okabe S, Tauchi T, Tanaka Y, et al. Efficacy of the dual PI3K and mTOR inhibitor NVP-BEZ235 in combination with nilotinib against BCR-ABL-positive leukemia cells involves the ABL kinase domain mutation. Cancer Biol Ther 2014;15: 207–15.

62. Chu S, Holtz M, Gupta M, et al. BCR/ABL kinase inhibition by imatinib mesylate enhances MAP kinase activity in chronic myelogenous leukemia CD34+ cells. Blood 2004;103:3167–74.

63. Ma L, Shan Y, Bai R, et al. A therapeutically targetable mechanism of BCR-ABL-independent imatinib resistance in chronic myeloid leukemia. Sci Transl Med 2014;6:252ra121.

64. Packer LM, Rana S, Hayward R, et al. Nilotinib and MEK inhibitors induce synthetic lethality through paradoxical activation of RAF in drug-resistant chronic myeloid leukemia. Cancer Cell 2011;20:715–27.

65. Asmussen J, Lasater EA, Tajon C, et al. MEK-dependent negative feedback underlies BCR-ABL-mediated oncogene addiction. Cancer Discov 2014;4:200–15.

66. Khorashad JS, Eiring AM, Mason CC, et al. shRNA library screening identifies nucleocytoplasmic transport as a mediator of BCR-ABL1 kinase-independent resistance. Blood 2015;125:1772–81.

67. Walker CJ, Oaks JJ, Santhanam R, et al. Preclinical and clinical efficacy of XPO1/CRM1 inhibition by the karyopherin inhibitor KPT-330 in Ph+ leukemias. Blood 2013;122:3034–44.

68. Scott MT, Korfi K, Saffrey P, et al. Epigenetic reprogramming sensitizes CML stem cells to combined EZH2 and tyrosine kinase inhibition. Cancer Discov 2016;6(11):1248–57.

69. Xie H, Peng C, Huang J, et al. Chronic myelogenous leukemia initiating cells require Polycomb group protein EZH2. Cancer Discov 2016;6(11):1237–47.

70. Zhang B, Li M, McDonald T, et al. Microenvironmental protection of CML stem and progenitor cells from tyrosine kinase inhibitors through N-cadherin and Wnt-beta-catenin signaling. Blood 2013;121:1824–38.

71. Ge X, Wang X. Role of Wnt canonical pathway in hematological malignancies. J Hematol Oncol 2010;3:33.

72. Zhao C, Blum J, Chen A, et al. Loss of beta-catenin impairs the renewal of normal and CML stem cells in vivo. Cancer Cell 2007;12:528–41.

73. Lim S, Saw TY, Zhang M, et al. Targeting of the MNK-eIF4E axis in blast crisis chronic myeloid leukemia inhibits leukemia stem cell function. Proc Natl Acad Sci U S A 2013;110:E2298–307.

74. Wu J, Meng F, Lu H, et al. Lyn regulates BCR-ABL and Gab2 tyrosine phosphorylation and c-Cbl protein stability in imatinib-resistant chronic myelogenous leukemia cells. Blood 2008;111:3821–9.

75. Wu J, Meng F, Kong LY, et al. Association between imatinib-resistant BCR-ABL mutation-negative leukemia and persistent activation of LYN kinase. J Natl Cancer Inst 2008;100:926–39.

76. Donato NJ, Wu JY, Stapley J, et al. BCR-ABL independence and LYN kinase overexpression in chronic myelogenous leukemia cells selected for resistance to STI571. Blood 2003;101:690–8.

77. O'Hare T, Eide CA, Deininger MW. Persistent LYN signaling in imatinib-resistant, BCR-ABL-independent chronic myelogenous leukemia. J Natl Cancer Inst 2008; 100:908–9.

78. Ng KP, Manjeri A, Lee KL, et al. Physiologic hypoxia promotes maintenance of CML stem cells despite effective BCR-ABL1 inhibition. Blood 2014;123:3316–26.

79. Irvine DA, Zhang B, Kinstrie R, et al. Deregulated hedgehog pathway signaling is inhibited by the smoothened antagonist LDE225 (Sonidegib) in chronic phase chronic myeloid leukaemia. Sci Rep 2016;6:25476.

80. Wu L, Yu J, Chen R, et al. Dual inhibition of Bcr-Abl and Hsp90 by C086 potently inhibits the proliferation of imatinib-resistant CML cells. Clin Cancer Res 2015; 21:833–43.

81. Kobayashi CI, Takubo K, Kobayashi H, et al. The IL-2/CD25 axis maintains distinct subsets of chronic myeloid leukemia-initiating cells. Blood 2014;123: 2540–9.

82. Chen Y, Peng C, Abraham SA, et al. Arachidonate 15-lipoxygenase is required for chronic myeloid leukemia stem cell survival. J Clin Invest 2014;124:3847–62.

83. Zhang B, Li L, Chen CC, et al. Knockdown (KD) of Mir-126 expression enhances tyrosine kinase inhibitor (TKI)-mediated targeting of chronic myelogenous leukemia (CML) stem cells. Blood 2015;126:51.

84. Dierks C, Beigi R, Guo GR, et al. Expansion of Bcr-Abl-positive leukemic stem cells is dependent on Hedgehog pathway activation. Cancer Cell 2008;14: 238–49.

85. Chen Y, Hu Y, Zhang H, et al. Loss of the Alox5 gene impairs leukemia stem cells and prevents chronic myeloid leukemia. Nat Genet 2009;41:783–92.

86. Neviani P, Harb JG, Oaks JJ, et al. PP2A-activating drugs selectively eradicate TKI-resistant chronic myeloid leukemic stem cells. J Clin Invest 2013;123: 4144–57.

87. Cramer-Morales K, Nieborowska-Skorska M, Scheibner K, et al. Personalized synthetic lethality induced by targeting RAD52 in leukemias identified by gene mutation and expression profile. Blood 2013;122:1293–304.

88. Peng C, Brain J, Hu Y, et al. Inhibition of heat shock protein 90 prolongs survival of mice with BCR-ABL-T315I-induced leukemia and suppresses leukemic stem cells. Blood 2007;110:678–85.

89. Li L, Wang L, Li L, et al. Activation of p53 by SIRT1 inhibition enhances elimination of CML leukemia stem cells in combination with imatinib. Cancer Cell 2012; 21:266–81.

90. Bellodi C, Lidonnici MR, Hamilton A, et al. Targeting autophagy potentiates tyrosine kinase inhibitor-induced cell death in Philadelphia chromosome-positive cells, including primary CML stem cells. J Clin Invest 2009;119:1109–23.

91. Ito K, Bernardi R, Morotti A, et al. PML targeting eradicates quiescent leukaemia-initiating cells. Nature 2008;453:1072–8.

92. Huang W, Luan CH, Hjort EE, et al. The role of Fas-associated phosphatase 1 in leukemia stem cell persistence during tyrosine kinase inhibitor treatment of chronic myeloid leukemia. Leukemia 2016;30:1502–9.

93. Jiang Q, Crews LA, Barrett CL, et al. ADAR1 promotes malignant progenitor reprogramming in chronic myeloid leukemia. Proc Natl Acad Sci U S A 2013;110: 1041–6.

94. Reavie L, Buckley SM, Loizou E, et al. Regulation of c-Myc ubiquitination controls chronic myelogenous leukemia initiation and progression. Cancer Cell 2013;23:362–75.

95. Abraham SA, Hopcroft LE, Carrick E, et al. Dual targeting of p53 and c-MYC selectively eliminates leukaemic stem cells. Nature 2016;534:341–6.

96. Hurtz C, Hatzi K, Cerchietti L, et al. BCL6-mediated repression of p53 is critical for leukemia stem cell survival in chronic myeloid leukemia. J Exp Med 2011; 208:2163–74.

97. Neviani P, Santhanam R, Oaks JJ, et al. FTY720, a new alternative for treating blast crisis chronic myelogenous leukemia and Philadelphia chromosome-positive acute lymphocytic leukemia. J Clin Invest 2007;117:2408–21.

98. Goff DJ, Court Recart A, Sadarangani A, et al. A Pan-BCL2 inhibitor renders bone-marrow-resident human leukemia stem cells sensitive to tyrosine kinase inhibition. Cell Stem Cell 2013;12:316–28.

99. Wylie A, Schoepfer J, Berellini G, et al. ABL001, a potent allosteric inhibitor of BCR-ABL, prevents emergence of resistant disease when administered in combination with nilotinib in an in vivo murine model of chronic myeloid leukemia. Blood 2014;124:398.

100. Ottmann OG, Alimena G, DeAngelo DJ, et al. ABL001, a potent, allosteric inhibitor of BCR-ABL, exhibits safety and promising single- agent activity in a phase I study of patients with CML with failure of prior TKI therapy. Blood 2015;126:138.

101. Smith BD, Hood MM, Kaufman MD, et al. Abstract B78: rebastinib, a small molecule TIE2 kinase inhibitor, prevents primary tumor growth and lung metastasis in the PyMT breast cancer model. Cancer Res 2013;73:B78.

102. Santos FP, Kantarjian H, Cortes J, et al. Bafetinib, a dual Bcr-Abl/Lyn tyrosine kinase inhibitor for the potential treatment of leukemia. Curr Opin Investig Drugs 2010;11:1450–65.

103. Borthakur G, Dombret H, Schafhausen P, et al. A phase I study of danusertib (PHA-739358) in adult patients with accelerated or blastic phase chronic myeloid leukemia and Philadelphia chromosome-positive acute lymphoblastic leukemia resistant or intolerant to imatinib and/or other second generation c-ABL therapy. Haematologica 2015;100:898–904.

104. Zabriskie MS, Eide CA, Yan D, et al. Extreme mutational selectivity of axitinib limits its potential use as a targeted therapeutic for BCR-ABL1-positive leukemia. Leukemia 2016;30:1418–21.

105. Pemovska T, Johnson E, Kontro M, et al. Axitinib effectively inhibits BCR-ABL1(T315I) with a distinct binding conformation. Nature 2015;519:102–5.

106. Kwak J-Y, Kim H, Kim JA, et al. Efficacy and safety of radotinib compared with imatinib in newly diagnosed chronic phase chronic myeloid leukemia patients: 12 months result of phase 3 clinical trial. Blood 2015;126:476.

107. Zabriskie MS, Vellore NA, Gantz KC, et al. Radotinib is an effective inhibitor of native and kinase domain-mutant BCR-ABL1. Leukemia 2015;29:1939–42.

108. Bhalla S, Tremblay D, Mascarenhas J. Discontinuing tyrosine kinase inhibitor therapy in chronic myelogenous leukemia: current understanding and future directions. Clin Lymphoma Myeloma Leuk 2016;16:488–94.

109. Saussele S, Richter J, Hochhaus A, et al. The concept of treatment-free remission in chronic myeloid leukemia. Leukemia 2016;30(8):1638–47.

110. Talpaz M, Hehlmann R, Quintas-Cardama A, et al. Re-emergence of interferon-alpha in the treatment of chronic myeloid leukemia. Leukemia 2013;27:803–12.

111. Preudhomme C, Guilhot J, Nicolini FE, et al. Imatinib plus peginterferon Alfa-2a in chronic myeloid leukemia. N Engl J Med 2010;363:2511–21.

112. Simonsson B, Gedde-Dahl T, Markevärn B, et al. Combination of pegylated IFN-α2b with imatinib increases molecular response rates in patients with low- or intermediate-risk chronic myeloid leukemia. Blood 2011;118:3228–35.

113. Hochhaus A, Saglio G, Hughes TP, et al. Long-term benefits and risks of frontline nilotinib vs imatinib for chronic myeloid leukemia in chronic phase: 5-year update of the randomized ENESTnd trial. Leukemia 2016;30:1044–54.

114. Hjorth-Hansen H, Stentoft J, Richter J, et al. Safety and efficacy of the combination of pegylated interferon-alpha2b and dasatinib in newly diagnosed chronic-phase chronic myeloid leukemia patients. Leukemia 2016;30:1853–60.

115. Nicolini FE, Etienne G, Dubruille V, et al. Nilotinib and peginterferon alfa-2a for newly diagnosed chronic-phase chronic myeloid leukaemia (NiloPeg): a

multicentre, non-randomised, open-label phase 2 study. Lancet Haematol 2015; 2:e37–46.

116. Roy L, Chomel JC, Guilhot J, et al. Combination of dasatinib and peg-interferon alpha 2b in chronic phase chronic myeloid leukemia (CP-CML) first line: preliminary results of a phase II trial, from the French Intergroup of CML (Fi-LMC). Blood 2015;126:134.

117. Cortes J, Saglio G, Baccarani M, et al. Final study results of the phase 3 dasatinib versus imatinib in newly diagnosed chronic myeloid leukemia in chronic phase (CML-CP) trial (DASISION, CA180-056). Blood 2014;124:152.

118. Pinilla-Ibarz J, Cathcart K, Korontsvit T, et al. Vaccination of patients with chronic myelogenous leukemia with bcr-abl oncogene breakpoint fusion peptides generates specific immune responses. Blood 2000;95:1781–7.

119. Bocchia M, Gentili S, Abruzzese E, et al. Effect of a p210 multipeptide vaccine associated with imatinib or interferon in patients with chronic myeloid leukaemia and persistent residual disease: a multicentre observational trial. Lancet 2005; 365:657–62.

120. Molldrem JJ, Lee PP, Wang C, et al. Evidence that specific T lymphocytes may participate in the elimination of chronic myelogenous leukemia. Nat Med 2000;6: 1018–23.

121. Rezvani K, Yong AS, Mielke S, et al. Repeated PR1 and WT1 peptide vaccination in Montanide-adjuvant fails to induce sustained high-avidity, epitope-specific CD8+ T cells in myeloid malignancies. Haematologica 2011;96:432–40.

122. Gao L, Bellantuono I, Elsasser A, et al. Selective elimination of leukemic CD34(+) progenitor cells by cytotoxic T lymphocytes specific for WT1. Blood 2000;95:2198–203.

123. Dubrovsky L, Pankov D, Brea EJ, et al. A TCR-mimic antibody to WT1 bypasses tyrosine kinase inhibitor resistance in human BCR-ABL+ leukemias. Blood 2014; 123:3296–304.

124. Järås M, Johnels P, Hansen N, et al. Isolation and killing of candidate chronic myeloid leukemia stem cells by antibody targeting of IL-1 receptor accessory protein. Proc Natl Acad Sci U S A 2010;107:16280–5.

125. Frolova O, Benito J, Brooks C, et al. SL-401 and SL-501, targeted therapeutics directed at the interleukin-3 receptor, inhibit the growth of leukaemic cells and stem cells in advanced phase chronic myeloid leukaemia. Br J Haematol 2014;166:862–74.

126. Lin H, Chen M, Rothe K, et al. Selective JAK2/ABL dual inhibition therapy effectively eliminates TKI-insensitive CML stem/progenitor cells. Oncotarget 2014;5: 8637–50.

127. Gallipoli P, Cook A, Rhodes S, et al. JAK2/STAT5 inhibition by nilotinib with ruxolitinib contributes to the elimination of CML CD34+ cells in vitro and in vivo. Blood 2014;124:1492–501.

128. Prost S, Relouzat F, Spentchian M, et al. Erosion of the chronic myeloid leukaemia stem cell pool by PPARgamma agonists. Nature 2015;525:380–3.

129. Huang X, Cortes J, Kantarjian H. Estimations of the increasing prevalence and plateau prevalence of chronic myeloid leukemia in the era of tyrosine kinase inhibitor therapy. Cancer 2012;118:3123–7.

The Development and Use of Janus Kinase 2 Inhibitors for the Treatment of Myeloproliferative Neoplasms

CrossMark

Gabriela S. Hobbs, MD[a,*,1], Sarah Rozelle, PhD[b,2],
Ann Mullally, MD[b,*,3]

KEYWORDS

- JAK2V617F mutation • Myeloproliferative neoplasms • JAK2 inhibitors
- JAK-STAT signaling • Myelofibrosis • Polycythemia vera • Mutant calreticulin

KEY POINTS

- Janus kinase (JAK) 2 inhibitors were developed as rationally designed therapy in myeloproliferative neoplasms (MPNs) following the discovery of the activating JAK2V617F mutation.
- The oral JAK1/JAK2 inhibitor ruxolitinib is approved by the Food and Drug Administration for the treatment of intermediate and advanced phase myelofibrosis and in certain cases of polycythemia vera.
- Activated JAK-signal transducer and activator of transcription (STAT) signaling is a central feature of MPN and, as a result, JAK2 inhibitors have clinical efficacy regardless of the type of MPN phenotypic driver mutation.
- Although providing clinical benefit to MPN patients, JAK2 inhibitors are not strongly clonally selective for either JAK2V617F-mutant or *CALR*-mutant MPN cells.
- Despite an absence of clonal selectivity for MPN cells and no difference in the rate of leukemic transformation, ruxolitinib seems to improve overall survival in myelofibrosis.

Disclosure Statement: The authors have no conflicts of interest.
[a] Division of Hematology/Oncology, Massachusetts General Hospital, Harvard Medical School, Boston, MA 02115, USA; [b] Division of Hematology, Department of Medicine, Brigham and Women's Hospital, Harvard Medical School, Boston, MA 02115, USA
[1] Present address: 100 Blossom Street Cox-1, Suite 110, Boston, MA 02114.
[2] Present address: Harvard Institutes of Medicine Building, 7th floor, 77 Avenue Louis Pasteur, Boston, MA 02115.
[3] Present address: Harvard Institutes of Medicine Building, Room 738, 77 Avenue Louis Pasteur, Boston, MA 02115.
* Corresponding authors.
E-mail addresses: ghobbs@partners.org (G.S.H.); amullally@partners.org (A.M.)

INTRODUCTION

The discovery of the JAK2V617F mutation in patients with myeloproliferative neo-plasms (MPNs) launched a new era of rationally designed molecularly targeted ther-apy in BCR-ABL negative MPN. The JAK2V617F mutation, which activates Janus kinase (JAK)-2 signaling, is present in more than 95% of patients with polycythemia vera (PV), approximately 65% of patients with myelofibrosis (MF), and 55% of pa-tients with essential thrombocythemia (ET).[1] Improved understanding of the molecu-lar biology of MPN has established activated JAK-signal transducer and activator of transcription (STAT) signaling, driven by JAK2V617F, MPLW515L/K, or mutant calre-ticulin (CALR) at the center of MPN pathogenesis,[2] establishing the JAK-STAT pathway as a key therapeutic target in these diseases (**Fig. 1**). The thrombopoietin receptor, MPL is mutated in between 1% and 5% of MPN cases, leading to cytokine independent growth and activated JAK-STAT signaling.[3] More recently, somatic mu-tations were discovered in the gene calreticulin (CALR) in 20% to 25% of ET and MF patients.[4,5] Calreticulin is a calcium-binding chaperone protein that localizes to the endoplasmic reticulum (ER) under normal conditions. More than 30 different

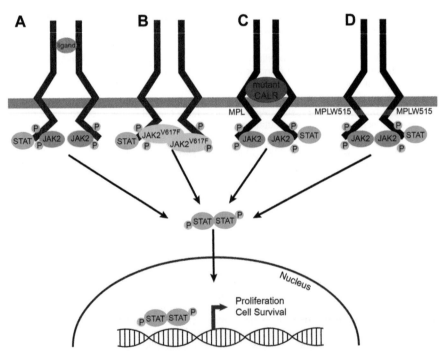

Fig. 1. JAK2-STAT signaling pathway activation in MPN. (A) Normally, JAK2-STAT signaling pathway activation occurs through ligand binding to and active dimerization of type 1 cyto-kine receptors (eg, MPL, EPOR, or GM-CSFR). Activated STAT translocates to the nucleus, where it binds promoters upregulating proliferation and cell survival genes. (B) The acti-vating mutation V617F in JAK2 leads to constitutive activation of JAK2-signaling indepen-dent of ligand binding. (C) Mutant CALR physically interacts with MPL to activate the MPL signaling pathway in a thrombopoietin-independent manner. (D) Mutation to MPL at amino acid 515 causes constitutively active MPL signaling. Note: Purple receptor denotes any type 1 cytokine receptor; blue receptors denote MPL.

mutations in *CALR* have been identified and all result in a +1 base pair frameshift that leads to the generation of a new C-terminal peptide in the mutant CALR protein that lacks the KDEL ER retention signal. Recent work has demonstrated that mutant CALR activates JAK-STAT signaling through physical interaction with MPL[6-9] consistent with the observation that *JAK2*, *MPL*, and *CALR* mutations are typically mutually exclusive in MPN.[5]

In addition to the 3 main MPN phenotype driver mutations, a few other mutations have been identified that also activate JAK-STAT signaling. For example, mutations in negative regulators of *JAK2*, such as *CBL*[10] and *LNK*,[11,12] have been described. There is also a small group of patients without identifiable MPN phenotype driver mutations, the so called triple-negative patients, and additional germline and somatic mutations in *JAK2* or *MPL* were recently identified in approximately 19% of these cases.[13]

Following the discovery of the JAK2V617F mutation in 2005, JAK2 inhibitors were rapidly developed and, in 2011, the Food and Drug Administration (FDA) approved the oral JAK1/2 inhibitor ruxolitinib for the treatment of intermediate and advanced phase MF. Since then, several other JAK inhibitors have entered advanced phase clinical trials. This article discusses the development and use of JAK inhibitors in MPN over the past decade.

PRECLINICAL DEVELOPMENT OF JANUS KINASE INHIBITORS

Following the discovery of the JAK2V617F mutation, the effects of the mutation on hematopoiesis were quickly modeled in mice. Using a retroviral bone marrow transplant (BMT) model, it was shown that JAK2V617F alone was sufficient to engender MPN in mice,[14] thus validating the mutation as a key molecular target in MPN. In parallel, JAK2 inhibitors were rapidly developed by several pharmaceutical companies and were soon shown to be safe and efficacious in the treatment of JAK2V617F-driven MPN in mice[15,16] and, subsequently, in MPLW515L retroviral BMT MPN mouse models.[17,18] Later, using a genetic Jak2V617F knockin mouse model, it was demonstrated that JAK2 inhibitors, although effective at reducing blood counts and splenomegaly, did not effectively target disease-propagating MPN stem cells,[19] a finding that was subsequently validated in clinical trials, in which JAK2 inhibitors have been disappointing in their ability to induce molecular remissions in MPN subjects.[20] More recently, the JAK inhibitor ruxolitinib was demonstrated to be efficacious in a transgenic model of mutant CALR,[21] although effects on mutant CALR allele burden were not measured. Genetic knockout of Jak2 in a retroviral MPLW515L MPN mouse model was shown to be superior to JAK2 inhibitor treatment,[22] suggesting that more potent JAK2 inhibition could enhance clinical efficacy in MPN patients. However, JAK2 signaling is also required for normal hematopoietic stem cell (HSC) function, as shown in a series of studies in which severe cell-intrinsic defects in HSC function, impaired hematopoiesis, and reduced survival were demonstrated following hematopoietic-specific conditional genetic deletion of Jak2 in adult mice.[23-25] These results have raised concerns regarding the potential for on-target hematological toxicity from more potent JAK2 inhibitors and reinforced efforts to develop JAK2V617F mutant-specific inhibitors. Combining ruxolitinib therapy with heat shock protein 90 (HSP90) inhibition was also shown to be efficacious in preclinical MPN mouse models.[26] This resulted in a phase II clinical trial of the HSP90 inhibitor, AUY922 in subjects with MF, which was terminated early due to excess gastrointestinal toxicity.[27] However, despite the toxicity, all 6 subjects treated in the trial experienced at least a partial response and 1 subject remained on study for longer than 1 year.

CLINICAL DEVELOPMENT OF JANUS KINASE INHIBITORS
Ruxolitinib for Myelofibrosis

Ruxolitinib is a JAK1/2 inhibitor approved for use in patients with intermediate-II and high risk MF. Ruxolitinib was approved based on 2 randomized phase III studies: Controlled Myelofibrosis Study with Oral JAK Inhibitor Treatment (COMFORT) I and II. COMFORT I compared ruxolitinib to placebo[28] and COMFORT II compared ruxolitinib it to best available therapy (BAT).[29] The primary endpoint of these studies was spleen volume reduction of greater than or equal to 35% at 24 weeks for the COMFORT I study and at 48 weeks for the COMFORT II study. Secondary endpoints included durability of response, improvement in symptoms as measured by the MF symptom assessment form (SAF), and overall survival.

In both studies, ruxolitinib led to durable symptom and spleen volume reduction. The MPN SAF total symptom score (TSS) was used to monitor changes in symptoms in the COMFORT I study.[30] In the COMFORT II study, several quality of life and symptom measurement tools were used, including the European Organization for Research and Treatment of Cancer (EORTC) quality-of life questionnaire core model (QLQ-C30) and the Functional Assessment of Cancer Therapy-Lymphoma (FACT-Lym) scale. In COMFORT I, 45.9% of subjects experienced a greater than 50% improvement in the MPN SAF TSS at 24 weeks, compared with 5.3% of subjects receiving placebo in COMFORT I. Significant and consistent improvements in symptoms were also found in the COMFORT II study in subjects receiving ruxolitinib compared with worsening symptoms in subjects receiving best available therapy (BAT).[29] Based on the remarkable benefit of ruxolitinib in alleviating MF-related symptoms, the revised International Working Group (IWG) for Myelofibrosis Research and Treatment and the European LeukemiaNet incorporated the term "clinical improvement" to the response criteria.[31]

Three-year pooled follow-up of these studies has shown a statistically significant improvement in overall survival.[32] Five-year pooled follow-up of the COMFORT II study showed that, among patients achieving a greater than or equal to 35% spleen volume reduction, the probability of maintaining response was 0.48 (95% confidence interval, 0.35–0.60) at 5 years (median 3.2 years). The median overall survival was not reached in ruxolitinib treated subjects and was 4.1 years in BAT subjects. No new adverse events were reported with longer follow-up.[33]

At the final 5-year follow-up of the COMFORT studies, the mean spleen volume reduction for subjects who remained on ruxolitinib was 37.6% at 264 weeks, at this time 18.5% of subjects randomized to ruxolitinib maintained a greater than or equal to 35% reduction in spleen volume compared with baseline. Median duration of this response was 168.3 weeks.[33]

The most common toxicities hematologic toxicities of ruxolitinib are thrombocytopenia and anemia. The initial drop in platelets and hemoglobin is generally most pronounced in the first month of therapy and improves or stabilizes thereafter. The starting dose for ruxolitinib is based on platelet count. Subjects with a platelet count of greater than 200×10^9/L start at 20 mg twice a day, those with platelets between 100 to 200×10^9/L start at 15 mg twice a day, and those with platelets between 50 to 99×10^9/L start at 5 mg twice a day. Ruxolitinib is not recommended for patients with lower platelet values. Ruxolitinib dosing should not be adjusted in the first 4 weeks of therapy and, thereafter, not more often than every 2 weeks.[34]

The most common nonhematologic adverse events reported in patients using ruxolitinib, include diarrhea and peripheral edema, but these were minor. Of particular concern are the potential infectious complications associated with ruxolitinib because this drug is immunosuppressive. In COMFORT I, herpes zoster occurred in 10.3% of subjects randomized to ruxolitinib and 13.5% of subjects who crossed over to ruxolitinib treatment.[35] In COMFORT II, the rates of urinary tract infection were 24.6%, pneumonia, 13.1%; herpes zoster reactivation, 11.5%; sepsis, 7.9%; and tuberculosis 1%.[33] In addition, there was 1 report of progressive multifocal leukoencephalopathy[36] and a case of cytomegalovirus retinitis.[37]

Based on the rarity of nonhematologic events, cytopenias are undoubtedly the most common reason for treatment discontinuation and limit which patients can initiate this drug. A recent study demonstrating that Jak2 is not required for terminal megakaryopoiesis and platelet production in mice suggests that ruxolitinib-related thrombocytopenia may occur as a result of JAK-STAT inhibition upstream in the hematopoietic hierarchy, namely in stem and/or progenitor cells, rather than in megakaryocytes and platelets.[38]

Another significant concern with ruxolitinib use is the potential for rapid rebound of symptoms and splenomegaly on discontinuation. This is of particular concern in patients who are approaching transplantation as optimal timing or necessity of discontinuation before transplant remains unknown. However, a trial is planned to address the feasibility of maintaining subjects on ruxolitinib during the conditioning and early pretransplant period to address this issue.

Although ruxolitinib represents a major treatment advance for patients with MF, this drug is associated with a high discontinuation rate mainly due to loss of efficacy and cytopenias.[39,40] In addition, ruxolitinib does not seem to alter the disease biology of MF and leads to small changes in JAK2V617F allele burden and in bone marrow fibrosis. A recent analysis of patients on ruxolitinib revealed that, of the 236 JAK2V617F mutant subjects in the COMFORT studies, only 20 subjects achieved partial and 6 subjects achieved complete molecular remissions, with a median time to respond of 22.2 and 27.5 months, respectively.[20] Moreover, ruxolitinib does not eliminate risk of progression to acute leukemia. Long-term follow-up from the COMFORT II study shows similar rates of progression to acute leukemia in ruxolitinib-treated subjects compared with those who received BAT.[33]

It should be noted that ruxolitinib is efficacious for MF patients regardless of their MPN phenotypic driver mutational status because activated JAK-STAT signaling is a common feature of MPN and ruxolitinib is not a JAK2V617F mutant-specific inhibitor. However, JAK-STAT inhibition in normal hematopoietic cells also explains some of the on-target toxicity of ruxolitinib; for example, anemia.

There has been a lot of speculation about why ruxolitinib is associated with a survival advantage despite its lack of clonal selectivity for JAK2V617F-mutant or CALR-mutant cells and its limited disease-modifying activity. Ruxolitinib is associated with a reduction in circulating cytokines[41] that may be responsible for the reduction in symptoms and spleen size. This in turn leads to improvement in functional status, which may then lead to improved outcomes. It is unclear if ruxolitinib has additional effects on halting disease progression through other as yet undefined mechanisms. Notably, the use of historical control cohorts for survival analysis comparisons has not helped in trying to clarify this issue.[42] The advantages and disadvantages of ruxolitinib in the treatment of MF are summarized in **Fig. 2** and ongoing studies are summarized in **Table 1**.

Finally, in addition to its use in MF, ruxolitinib was approved for use in patients with PV who were resistant or intolerant to therapy with hydroxyurea.[43]

Ruxolitinib for Polycythemia Vera

In 2014, ruxolitinib was approved for PV based on the results of the REPSONSE phase III study.[43] This study compared ruxolitinib (10 mg twice daily) with BAT in patients with

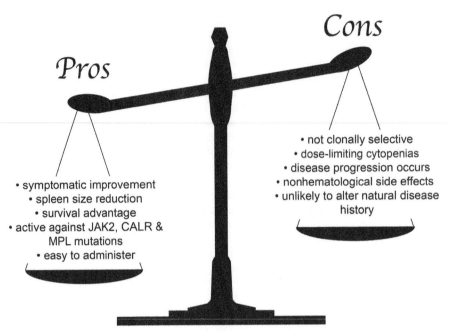

Pros

• symptomatic improvement
• spleen size reduction
• survival advantage
• active against JAK2, CALR & MPL mutations
• easy to administer

Cons

• not clonally selective
• dose-limiting cytopenias
• disease progression occurs
• nonhematological side effects
• unlikely to alter natural disease history

Fig. 2. Summary of the pros and cons of JAK2 inhibitor treatment in MPN patients.

PV who were unable to take hydroxyurea due to intolerance or lack of response. The primary endpoints of this study were hematocrit control and spleen volume reduction of greater than or equal to 35% at 32 weeks. The secondary endpoints included the proportion of subjects who maintained response at 48 weeks and achievement of complete hematologic remission at 32 weeks. A total of 222 subjects were enrolled and 21% of subjects achieved the primary endpoint versus less than 1% for BAT. Most subjects (77%) reached at least 1 component of the composite primary endpoint by week 32. Ruxolitinib was also associated with significant improvements in symptoms based on the MPN SAF.[44] In general, ruxolitinib was well tolerated with few adverse hematologic events. Herpes zoster virus infection was seen in 6.4% of ruxolitinib-treated subjects versus 0% of BAT-treated subjects. Long-term follow-up on the RESPONSE study is awaited. In addition, a separate phase III study evaluating the efficacy and feasibility of frontline ruxolitinib therapy in high-risk PV and ET subjects is ongoing (Ruxo-BEAT trial, clinicaltrials.gov, NCT02577926).

Pacritinib

Pacritinib (SB1518) is a JAK2, FMS-like tyrosine kinase 3 (FLT3), IRAK1, and CFSR1 inhibitor that is in advanced clinical testing. The development of pacritinib was interrupted due to an FDA hold that was lifted earlier this year. In August 2014, pacritinib received fast-track designation by the FDA. Unfortunately, based on reports of patient deaths secondary to intracranial hemorrhage, cardiac failure, and cardiac arrest in the PERSIST-2 trial, the FDA placed pacritinib on a clinical hold. At that point, CTI Bio-Pharma withdrew its new drug application; however, the FDA allowed subjects who were receiving benefit from pacritinib at the time of the clinical hold to remain on the drug.

Table 1
Ongoing studies using ruxolitinib for myelofibrosis

Drug	Drug Class	Phase	Trial	Primary Endpoint
Studies with ruxolitinib				
Ruxolitinib	JAK1/2 inhibitor	IB	NCT01317875	Determine dose for MF patients with platelets $<100 \times 10^9$/L
		II	NCT01795677	Before allogeneic transplant safety or efficacy
		III	NCT02598297	Early MF with high-risk mutations
		I–II	NCT02806375	With post-transplant cyclophosphamide in subjects with MF
		II–III	NCT02962388	ET-ruxolitinib vs BAT failure-free time
		III	NCT02962388	ET and PV-ruxolitinib vs BAT efficacy
Combination studies				
Ruxolitinib + INCB050465	PI3K-delta inhibitor	II	NCT02718300	Safety or efficacy
Ruxolitinib + TGR-1202	PI3 kinase inhibitor	I	NCT02493530	DLT, safety
Ruxolitinib + Idelalisib	PI3K delta kinase inhibitor	IB	NCT02436135	DLT, safety
Ruxolitinib + Vismodegib	Hedgehog inhibitor	I–II	NCT02593760	Efficacy
Ruxolitinib + PIM447	PIM inhibitor	IB	NCT02370706	DLT, safety
Ruxolitinib + Glasdegib	Hedgehog pathway inhibitor	II	NCT02226172	Safety, efficacy
Ruxolitinib and Decitabine	Hypomethylating agent	I–II	NCT02076191	MTD, safety efficacy
Ruxolitinib and Azacitidine	Hypomethylating agent	II	NCT01787487	Efficacy
Ruxolitinib + Pracinostat	HDAC inhibitor	II	NCT03069326	Efficacy, tolerability
Ruxolitinib + Peg-Interferon Alpha-2a	Interferon	I–II	NCT02742324	Safety, efficacy
Ruxolitinib + Sotatercept	Soluble activin receptor type wA IgG-FC fusion protein	II	NCT01712308	Anemia response
Thalidomide	Immunomodulatory agent	II	NCT03069326	Efficacy
Pomalidomide	Immunomodulatory agent	IB–II	NCT01644110	Efficacy
Idelalisib	PI3Kδ inhibitor	I	NCT02436135	Safety

Abbreviations: DLT, dose limiting toxicity; HDAC, histone deacetylase; MTD, maximum tolerated dose; PIM, Proviral Integrations of Moloney virus (PIM) serine/threonine kinase.

Pacritinib, like ruxolitinib, inhibits JAK2 signaling and is, therefore, efficacious regardless of the patient's JAK2V617F mutational status. In addition, pacritinib does not inhibit other JAK family kinases for example, JAK1, as potently as ruxolitinib, resulting in an altered side effect profile compared with ruxolitinib. Studies with pacritinib have allowed subjects to enroll regardless of cytopenias and some subjects in these studies have experienced improvements in blood counts, potentially due to differential effects of pacritinib on cytokine signaling as compared with ruxolitinib. A kinome analysis determined that, unlike ruxolitinib, pacritinib inhibits JAK2 but not JAK1 and that pacritinib also inhibits interleukin-1 receptor-associated kinase 1, which may explain its capacity for improving constitutional symptoms.[45] In addition, like ruxolitinib, pacritinib leads to reductions in splenomegaly.[46,47]

Pacritinib is undergoing phase III testing in the PERSIST-1 (NCT01773187) and PERSIST-2 (NCT02055781) studies. The primary endpoint for both studies is the proportion of subjects achieving greater than or equal to 35% reduction in spleen volume at week 24 by MRI. PERSIST-1 compared the efficacy and safety of pacritinib 400 mg daily with BAT in subjects with intermediate-1 or higher primary and secondary MF.[48] Subjects treated with pacritinib experienced improvement in symptoms regardless of subjects characteristics.[49] Spleen volume reduction rates at week 24 were 19.1% for pacritinib versus 4.7% of BAT in the intent-to-treat group. Overall, pacritinib was well-tolerated with diarrhea, nausea, and vomiting as the most common adverse events. Approximately 300 subjects were enrolled in PERSIST-2, which compared the efficacy and safety of 2 dosing schedules, 200 mg twice daily and 400 mg daily, compared with BAT in subjects with thrombocytopenia ($\leq$100,000/μL).

The results of PERSIST-2 were recently presented at the American Society of Hematology (ASH) Annual Meeting in 2016 as a late-breaking abstract.[50] The results of the study were promising, particularly because subjects with cytopenias and subjects who had previously received ruxolitinib derived a benefit from this drug. Of the subjects on the study, a significant percentage had received ruxolitinib at some point in their therapy (44%). In terms of efficacy, 18% of pacritinib-treated subjects achieved a greater than or equal to 35% spleen volume reduction compared with 3% in the BAT arm; 32% of subjects in the pacritinib arm achieved a greater than or equal to 50% reduction in symptoms versus 14% in the BAT arm. In addition, 19% of subjects in the pacritinib once-daily dosing arm and 22% in the twice a day dosing arm reduced their red cell transfusion dependence at week 24 compared with 9% in the BAT arm. There was no significant difference in overall survival for either treatment dose. The most common toxicities associated with pacritinib were gastrointestinal and cytopenias. The investigators reported bleeding and cardiac toxicities, although it was not specified if these occurred more frequently in the pacritinib-treated arm compared with BAT. However, grade 3 or 4 bleeding was more common in patients with grade 3-4 thrombocytopenia, which occurred more frequently in the pacritinib twice a day group. One subject in the pacritinib daily group had intracranial hemorrhage and there were none in the other groups. Results from these studies have allowed pacritinib to continue in clinical development and the FDA lifted its hold in January 2017.

Momelotinib

Momelotinib (CYT387) is a JAK1/2 inhibitor that is currently undergoing phase III testing. The phase I-II study included patients with intermediate or high-risk primary or secondary MF. Anemia and spleen responses were noted in 59% and 48%, respectively, per IWG criteria, 70% of transfusion-dependent subjects achieved transfusion independence, 39% experienced reduction in spleen size, and greater than 50% experienced improvement in symptoms. Grade 3-4 thrombocytopenia developed in

32% of recipients.[51] A follow-up study, reported that 58 of 120 subjects remained on treatment with a median treatment duration of 507 days (range 23–1036). Median duration of spleen response was 324 days (range 56–936 days), median duration of anemia response was not yet reached (57–987 days), and a significant percentage of subjects reported improvement in constitutional symptoms.[51]

Results of the momelotinib phase I-II studies were updated at the ASH conference in 2016. This study was a sponsor-independent report with 6-year follow-up with a median of 3.2 years of follow-up. At this point, 88 subjects had discontinued the drug and 70 had died, 12 subjects remain on study, and 5 have received a stem cell transplant. As with the prior reports, the most common adverse events included cytopenias. Almost half of the subjects developed grade 1 or 2 neuropathy, which was not reversible. Clinical improvement occurred in 57% of subjects, 44% had an anemia response, 51% of transfusion-dependent subjects became transfusion-independent, and 43% had a spleen response.[52]

There are 2 ongoing phase III studies. SIMPLIFY-1 (NCT01969838) is a double-blind, active-controlled study for subjects with primary or secondary intermediate-risk and high-risk MF who are naive to JAK2 therapy, comparing ruxolitinib versus momelotinib; 420 subjects will be enrolled. SIMPLIFY-2 (NCT02101268) is a randomized, open-label study that will evaluate the efficacy of momelotinib versus BAT in subjects with anemia or thrombocytopenia with primary or secondary MF previously treated with ruxolitinib.

NS-018

NS-018 is a selective JAK2 inhibitor, with less activity against other JAK family kinases. Results of the phase I-II study in intermediate-1 or higher risk patients with primary or secondary MF were presented at the ASH meeting in 2016.[53] Forty-eight subjects were enrolled across 10 dosing cohorts, 10 subjects currently remain on treatment. Of the subjects treated, 29 had received prior JAK inhibitor therapy. In the phase I study,[54] 37% of subjects experienced reduction in bone marrow fibrosis of 1 or more; this was not reported in the phase II study. In all dose cohorts, greater than or equal to 50% of subjects experienced a greater than or equal to 50% reduction in MF-SAF score. Among 36 subjects with splenomegaly at enrollment, 20 showed a greater than or equal to 50% reduction in spleen size. The major adverse events seen were hematologic and nausea. Neurologic toxicity with peripheral neuropathy, headache, and dizziness were seen in the phase I portion of the study.

INCB-39100

Results of a phase II study of INCB-39110, a selective JAK1 inhibitor, have shown improvement in MF symptoms, as well as some improvement in splenomegaly.[55] Adverse events included fatigue, constipation, diarrhea, upper respiratory tract infection, cough, and nausea. Cytopenias were common; 33% of subjects developed worsening grade 3 anemia and 24% developed thrombocytopenia.

In addition to the JAK inhibitors previously mentioned, other JAK inhibitors have been evaluated that are no longer in development, including, BMS911543, gandotinib, and fedratinib.

FUTURE DIRECTIONS AND DEVELOPMENT OF MUTANT-SPECIFIC JAK2V617F INHIBITORS

A key goal in MPN therapy is to identify drugs that preferentially target MPN cells over normal cells and, in particular, drugs that selectively target MPN stem cells over normal HSC. Three potential approaches under investigation to achieve this goal are highlighted here.

Targeting Janus Kinase-2 in the Inactive State

Ruxolitinib and other JAK2 inhibitors currently in clinical trials target the adenosine triphosphate (ATP)-binding pocket of JAK2 and stabilize the active conformation of the kinase – so called, type 1 inhibition. Despite blocking kinase function, type 1 inhibitors can lead to an increase in JAK2 activation loop phosphorylation.[56] Recently, type 2 JAK inhibitors, which stabilize the inactive unphosphorylated conformation of JAK2, resulting in more potent JAK2 inhibition, were reported. In addition to binding the ATP pocket, type 2 inhibitors bind supplemental adjacent sites, thus enhancing their specificity. The type 2 JAK inhibitor, CHZ868 (Novartis), was shown to be active in both in vitro and in vivo models of MPN and was found to preferentially target Jak2V617F cells over Jak2 wild-type cells in Jak2V617F mice.[57] Because type 2 inhibitors also bind wild-type Jak2, the preferential targeting of Jak2V617F cells may be a result of their increased proliferative rate compared with wild-type cells.

Targeting the Adenosine Triphosphate Binding Site in the Janus Kinase-2 Pseudokinase Domain

The JAK2 pseudokinase domain, in which the V617F mutation occurs, has been shown to bind ATP. Importantly, this binding seems to be differentially required for the kinase activity of JAK2V617F compared with wild-type JAK2, suggesting an avenue for mutant-specific JAK2 inhibition. To date, no ATP-competitive inhibitors that bind the JAK2 pseudokinase domain have been described but the pseudokinase domains of the other JAK family members, TYK2 and JAK1, have been shown to bind both ATP and ATP-competitive inhibitors. Furthermore, TYK2 signaling inhibition has been demonstrated using 1 of the compounds, providing proof-of-concept for this approach as a means to inhibit JAK pathway signaling.[58]

Targeting Allosteric Sites Specifically Involved in JAK2V617F Activation

A recent series of biochemical studies have advanced the understanding of the requirements for the JAK2V617F-driven activation and identified specific residues that could potentially be targeted with allosteric small molecule inhibitors.[59]

Summary

In the 12 years since the discovery of the JAK2V617F mutation in 2005, MPN research has been invigorated and very active. Consequentially, a tremendous amount of progress has been made over this time. Initially, it was hoped that inhibition of constitutively activated JAK2 signaling would lead to remissions in MPN that were akin to those seen in the treatment of chronic myelogenous leukemia (CML) with imatinib. Now, it is clear that the situation is more complex and the dependence on JAK2 signaling in MPN does not seem to be to the same degree as ABL kinase signaling dependence in CML. With recent advances in understanding the structural biology, biochemistry, and signaling activation of JAK2V617F, the development of JAK2V617F mutant-specific inhibitors seems attainable in the not too distant future. It remains to be seen if the next generation of JAK inhibitors, including mutant-specific JAK2 inhibitors, will be able to achieve more durable and meaningful remissions, not only improving symptoms but also achieving molecular remissions and altering the natural history of MPN.

ACKNOWLEDGMENTS

This work was supported by the NIH (R01HL131835 to AM; K12CA087723-14 to GSH), a Damon Runyon clinical investigator award (AM) and the Starr Cancer Consortium (AM).

REFERENCES

1. Levine RL, Wadleigh M, Cools J, et al. Activating mutation in the tyrosine kinase JAK2 in polycythemia vera, essential thrombocythemia, and myeloid metaplasia with myelofibrosis. Cancer Cell 2005;7(4):387–97.
2. Rampal R, Al-Shahrour F, Abdel-Wahab O, et al. Integrated genomic analysis illustrates the central role of JAK-STAT pathway activation in myeloproliferative neoplasm pathogenesis. Blood 2014;123(22):e123–33.
3. Pikman Y, Lee BH, Mercher T, et al. MPLW515L is a novel somatic activating mutation in myelofibrosis with myeloid metaplasia. PLoS Med 2006;3(7):e270.
4. Klampfl T, Gisslinger H, Harutyunyan AS, et al. Somatic mutations of calreticulin in myeloproliferative neoplasms. N Engl J Med 2013;369(25):2379–90.
5. Nangalia J, Massie CE, Baxter EJ, et al. Somatic CALR mutations in myeloproliferative neoplasms with nonmutated JAK2. N Engl J Med 2013;369(25):2391–405.
6. Araki M, Yang Y, Masubuchi N, et al. Activation of the thrombopoietin receptor by mutant calreticulin in CALR-mutant myeloproliferative neoplasms. Blood 2016; 127(10):1307–16.
7. Chachoua I, Pecquet C, El-Khoury M, et al. Thrombopoietin receptor activation by myeloproliferative neoplasm associated calreticulin mutants. Blood 2016; 127(10):1325–35.
8. Elf S, Abdelfattah NS, Chen E, et al. Mutant calreticulin requires both its mutant c-terminus and the thrombopoietin receptor for oncogenic transformation. Cancer Discov 2016;6(4):368–81.
9. Marty C, Pecquet C, Nivarthi H, et al. Calreticulin mutants in mice induce an MPL-dependent thrombocytosis with frequent progression to myelofibrosis. Blood 2016;127(10):1317–24.
10. Sanada M, Suzuki T, Shih LY, et al. Gain-of-function of mutated C-CBL tumour suppressor in myeloid neoplasms. Nature 2009;460(7257):904–8.
11. Grand FH, Hidalgo-Curtis CE, Ernst T, et al. Frequent CBL mutations associated with 11q acquired uniparental disomy in myeloproliferative neoplasms. Blood 2009;113(24):6182–92.
12. Oh ST, Simonds EF, Jones C, et al. Novel mutations in the inhibitory adaptor protein LNK drive JAK-STAT signaling in patients with myeloproliferative neoplasms. Blood 2010;116(6):988–92.
13. Milosevic Feenstra JD, Nivarthi H, Gisslinger H, et al. Whole-exome sequencing identifies novel MPL and JAK2 mutations in triple-negative myeloproliferative neoplasms. Blood 2016;127(3):325–32.
14. Wernig G, Mercher T, Okabe R, et al. Expression of Jak2V617F causes a polycythemia vera-like disease with associated myelofibrosis in a murine bone marrow transplant model. Blood 2006;107(11):4274–81.
15. Wernig G, Kharas MG, Okabe R, et al. Efficacy of TG101348, a selective JAK2 inhibitor, in treatment of a murine model of JAK2V617F-induced polycythemia vera. Cancer Cell 2008;13(4):311–20.
16. Tyner JW, Bumm TG, Deininger J, et al. CYT387, a novel JAK2 inhibitor, induces hematologic responses and normalizes inflammatory cytokines in murine myeloproliferative neoplasms. Blood 2010;115(25):5232–40.

17. Koppikar P, Abdel-Wahab O, Hedvat C, et al. Efficacy of the JAK2 inhibitor INCB16562 in a murine model of MPLW515L-induced thrombocytosis and myelofibrosis. Blood 2010;115(14):2919–27.

18. Wernig G, Kharas MG, Mullally A, et al. EXEL-8232, a small-molecule JAK2 inhibitor, effectively treats thrombocytosis and extramedullary hematopoiesis in a murine model of myeloproliferative neoplasm induced by MPLW515L. Leukemia 2012;26(4):720–7.

19. Mullally A, Lane SW, Ball B, et al. Physiological Jak2V617F expression causes a lethal myeloproliferative neoplasm with differential effects on hematopoietic stem and progenitor cells. Cancer Cell 2010;17(6):584–96.

20. Deininger M, Radich J, Burn TC, et al. The effect of long-term ruxolitinib treatment on JAK2p.V617F allele burden in patients with myelofibrosis. Blood 2015;126(13): 1551–4.

21. Shide K, Kameda T, Yamaji T, et al. Calreticulin mutant mice develop essential thrombocythemia that is ameliorated by the JAK inhibitor ruxolitinib. Leukemia 2017;31(5):1136–44.

22. Bhagwat N, Koppikar P, Keller M, et al. Improved targeting of JAK2 leads to increased therapeutic efficacy in myeloproliferative neoplasms. Blood 2014; 123(13):2075–83.

23. Park SO, Wamsley HL, Bae K, et al. Conditional deletion of Jak2 reveals an essential role in hematopoiesis throughout mouse ontogeny: implications for Jak2 inhibition in humans. PLoS One 2013;8(3):e59675.

24. Akada H, Akada S, Hutchison RE, et al. Critical role of Jak2 in the maintenance and function of adult hematopoietic stem cells. Stem Cells 2014;32(7):1878–89.

25. Grisouard J, Hao-Shen H, Dirnhofer S, et al. Selective deletion of Jak2 in adult mouse hematopoietic cells leads to lethal anemia and thrombocytopenia. Haematologica 2014;99(4):e52–4.

26. Marubayashi S, Koppikar P, Taldone T, et al. HSP90 is a therapeutic target in JAK2-dependent myeloproliferative neoplasms in mice and humans. J Clin Invest 2010;120(10):3578–93.

27. Hobbs G, Litvin R, Ahn J, et al. AUY922, a Heat Shock Protein 90 (Hsp90) Inhibitor, Demonstrates Activity in Patients with Myeloproliferative Neoplasms (MPNs). Blood 2015;126(23):4075.

28. Verstovsek S, Mesa RA, Gotlib J, et al. A double-blind, placebo-controlled trial of ruxolitinib for myelofibrosis. N Engl J Med 2012;366(9):799–807.

29. Harrison C, Kiladjian J-J, Al-Ali HK, et al. JAK inhibition with ruxolitinib versus best available therapy for myelofibrosis. N Engl J Med 2012;366(9):787–98.

30. Barbui T, Barosi G, Birgegard G, et al. Philadelphia-negative classical myeloproliferative neoplasms: critical concepts and management recommendations from European LeukemiaNet. J Clin Oncol 2011;29(6):761–70.

31. Tefferi A, Cervantes F, Mesa R, et al. Revised response criteria for myelofibrosis: International Working Group-Myeloproliferative Neoplasms Research and Treatment (IWG-MRT) and European LeukemiaNet (ELN) consensus report. Blood 2013;122(8):1395–8.

32. Hagop K, Kiladjian J-J, Gotlib J, et al. A Pooled Overall Survival Analysis of The COMFORT Studies: 2 Randomized Phase 3 Trials of Ruxolitinib For The Treatment of Myelofibrosis. Blood 2013;122(21):2820.

33. Harrison CN, Vannucchi AM, Kiladjian JJ, et al. Long-term findings from COMFORT-II, a phase 3 study of ruxolitinib vs best available therapy for myelofibrosis. Leukemia 2016;30(8):1701–7.

34. Mesa RA, Cortes J. Optimizing management of ruxolitinib in patients with myelo-fibrosis: the need for individualized dosing. J Hematol Oncol 2013;6:79.
35. Arana Yi C, Tam CS, Verstovsek S. Efficacy and safety of ruxolitinib in the treatment of patients with myelofibrosis. Future Oncol 2015;11(5):719–33.
36. Wathes R, Moule S, Milojkovic D. Progressive multifocal leukoencephalopathy associated with ruxolitinib. N Engl J Med 2013;369(2):197–8.
37. von Hofsten J, Johnsson Forsberg M, Zetterberg M. Cytomegalovirus retinitis in a patient who received ruxolitinib. N Engl J Med 2016;374(3):296–7.
38. Meyer SC, Keller MD, Woods BA, et al. Genetic studies reveal an unexpected negative regulatory role for Jak2 in thrombopoiesis. Blood 2014;124(14):2280–4.
39. Tefferi A, Litzow MR, Pardanani A. Long-term outcome of treatment with ruxolitinib in myelofibrosis. N Engl J Med 2011;365(15):1455–7.
40. Tefferi A, Pardanani A. Serious adverse events during ruxolitinib treatment discontinuation in patients with myelofibrosis. Mayo Clin Proc 2011;86(12):1188–91.
41. Verstovsek S, Kantarjian H, Mesa RA, et al. Safety and efficacy of INCB018424, a JAK1 and JAK2 inhibitor, in myelofibrosis. N Engl J Med 2010;363(12):1117–27.
42. Mascarenhas J, Hoffman R. A comprehensive review and analysis of the effect of ruxolitinib therapy on the survival of patients with myelofibrosis. Blood 2013;121(24):4832–7.
43. Vannucchi AM. Ruxolitinib versus standard therapy for the treatment of polycythemia vera. N Engl J Med 2015;372(17):1670–1.
44. Mesa R, Verstovsek S, Kiladjian JJ, et al. Changes in quality of life and disease-related symptoms in patients with polycythemia vera receiving ruxolitinib or standard therapy. Eur J Haematol 2016;97(2):192–200.
45. Singer JW, Al-Fayoumi S, Ma H, et al. Comprehensive kinase profile of pacritinib, a nonmyelosuppressive Janus kinase 2 inhibitor. J Exp Pharmacol 2016;8:11–9.
46. Komrokji R, Wadleigh M, Seymour JF, et al. Results of a phase 2 study of pacritinib (SB1518), a novel oral JAK2 inhibitor, in patients with primary, post-polycythemia vera, and post-essential thrombocythemia myelofibrosis. Blood 2011;118(21) [Abstract 282].
47. Komrokji RS, Seymour JF, Roberts AW, et al. Results of a phase 2 study of pacritinib (SB1518), a JAK2/JAK2(V617F) inhibitor, in patients with myelofibrosis. Blood 2015;125(17):2649–55.
48. Mesa R, Egyed M, Sxoke A, et al. Results of the PERSIST-1 phase III study of pacritinib (PAC) versus best available therapy (BAT) in primary myelofibrosis (PMF), post-polycythemia vera myelofibrosis (PPV-MF), or post-essential thrombocythemia-myelofibrosis (PET-MF). J Clin Oncol 2015;33(Suppl) [Abstract LBA7006].
49. Vannucchi AM, Mesa RA, Cervantes F, et al. Analysis of outcomes by patient subgroups in patients with myelofibrosis treated with pacritinib vs best available therapy (BAT) in the phase III persist-1 trial. Blood 2015;58.
50. Mascarenhas J, Hoffman R, Talpaz M, et al. Results of the persist-2 phase 3 study of pacritinib (PAC) versus best available therapy (BAT), including ruxolitinib (RUX), in patients (pts) with myelofibrosis (MF) and platelet counts <100,000/µl. Blood 2016;128(22). LBA-5-LBA-5.
51. Pardanani A, Laborde RR, Lasho TL, et al. Safety and efficacy of CYT387, a JAK1 and JAK2 inhibitor, in myelofibrosis. Leukemia 2013;27(6):1322–7.
52. Tefferi A, Barraco D, Lasho TL, et al. Momelotinib therapy in myelofibrosis: 6-years follow-up data on safety, efficacy and the impact of mutations on overall and relapse-free survival. Blood 2016;128(22):1123.

53. Verstovsek S, Talpaz M, Ritchie EK, et al. Phase 1/2 study of NS-018, an oral JAK2 inhibitor, in patients with primary myelofibrosis (PMF), post-polycythemia vera myelofibrosis (postPV MF), or post-essential thrombocythemia myelofibrosis (postET MF). Blood 2016;128(22):1936.

54. Verstovsek S, Talpaz M, Ricthie E, et al. A phase 1/2 Study of NS-018, an oral JAK2 inhibitor, in patients with primary myelofibrosis (PMF), post-polycythemia vera, myelofibrosis (pPV MF), or post-essential thrombocythemia myelofibrosis (pET MF). Blood 2015;126:2800.

55. Mascarenhas JO, Talpaz M, Gupta V, et al. Primary analysis results from an open-label phase II study of INCB039110, a selective JAK1 inhibitor, in patients with myelofibrosis. Blood 2014;124(21):714.

56. Andraos R, Qian Z, Bonenfant D, et al. Modulation of activation-loop phosphorylation by JAK inhibitors is binding mode dependent. Cancer Discov 2012;2(6):512–23.

57. Meyer SC, Keller MD, Chiu S, et al. CHZ868, a type II JAK2 inhibitor, reverses type I JAK inhibitor persistence and demonstrates efficacy in myeloproliferative neoplasms. Cancer Cell 2015;28(1):15–28.

58. Tokarski JS, Zupa-Fernandez A, Tredup JA, et al. tyrosine kinase 2-mediated signal transduction in T lymphocytes is blocked by pharmacological stabilization of its pseudokinase domain. J Biol Chem 2015;290(17):11061–74.

59. Leroy E, Dusa A, Colau D, et al. Uncoupling JAK2 V617F activation from cytokine-induced signalling by modulation of JH2 alphaC helix. Biochem J 2016;473(11):1579–91.

Mechanisms of Resistance to JAK2 Inhibitors in Myeloproliferative Neoplasms

 CrossMark

Sara C. Meyer, MD, PhD

KEYWORDS

• JAK2 • Myeloproliferative neoplasms • JAK2 inhibition • Resistance

KEY POINTS

• Resistance of myeloproliferative neoplasm (MPN) cells to JAK2 inhibitors develops based on reactivation of JAK-STAT signaling by JAK heterodimer formation, or protective cytokine effects.

• Acquired *JAK2* resistance mutations have not been observed in patients with MPN so far.

• JAK2 inhibitor–resistant MPN cells remain dependent on JAK2, consistent with incomplete target inhibition by the current type I JAK2 inhibitors.

• Resistance to the current type I JAK2 inhibitors like ruxolitinib is overcome by a novel type of JAK2 inhibition with an alternative binding mode (type II JAK2 inhibition), by HSP-90 inhibitors, or by combined pathway inhibition including Bcl-2/Bcl-xL, PI3K/Akt, or PIM kinase inhibition.

• Intermittent treatment with ruxolitinib could help to manage type I JAK2 inhibitor resistance, but may be complicated by potential flaring of symptoms on pausing ruxolitinib.

INTRODUCTION

Myeloproliferative neoplasms (MPNs) are chronic leukemias occurring at an annual incidence of 0.5 to 1.0 per 100,000.[1] They are hematopoietic stem cell disorders leading to excessive proliferation of mature myeloid cells. The 3 main MPN clinical phenotypes include essential thrombocythemia (ET) with marked thrombocytosis, polycythemia vera (PV) with erythrocytosis often along with neutrophilia and thrombocytosis, and myelofibrosis (MF) with expansion of megakaryocytes, progressive bone marrow fibrosis, and extramedullary hematopoiesis.[2] Splenomegaly and elevated serum cytokine levels are typical and contribute to symptom burden.[3] Myelofibrosis is the rarest (0.47/100,000 annually[1]) and most severe form of MPN with life expectancies limited to a few months in the presence of high-risk features.[4] MF transforms

Conflicts of interest: None.
Division of Hematology, Department of Biomedicine, University Hospital Basel, Hebelstrasse 20, Basel 4031, Switzerland
E-mail address: sara.meyer@unibas.ch

Hematol Oncol Clin N Am 31 (2017) 627–642
http://dx.doi.org/10.1016/j.hoc.2017.04.003
0889-8588/17/© 2017 Elsevier Inc. All rights reserved.

hemonc.theclinics.com

to secondary acute myeloid leukemia (AML) in 15% to 20% of patients (0.09/100,000 annually) with dismal prognosis or alternatively leads to hematopoietic failure. The sole curative therapy for MPN to date is hematopoietic stem cell transplantation. As MPNs mainly affect the elderly, only a limited subset of patients is eligible showing reduced success rates. Interferon-α has shown disease-modifying activity with molecular responses, but application is limited by poor tolerability.[2] Other therapies focus merely on symptom control and prevention of thromboembolic and hemorrhagic events complicating the disease, without altering the natural course of MPN.

The breakthrough discovery of the V617F gain-of-function mutation in the tyrosine kinase Janus kinase 2 (*JAK2*) in 2005 for the first time denominated a molecular therapeutic target.[5–8] *JAK2*V617F is present in 95% of PV and 50% to 60% of MF and ET. JAK2 is an intracellular non-receptor tyrosine kinase essential for hematopoiesis. It represents the exclusive mediator of cytokine signaling from the thrombopoietin receptor MPL, the erythropoietin and granulocyte-macrophage colony-stimulating factor receptors.[9,10] Hematopoietic cytokines binding to their cognate receptors induce JAK2 dimerization and phosphorylation.[11] Activated JAK2 initiates signaling through several intracellular signaling pathways, including the signal transducers and activators of transcription (STAT)3 and STAT5 transcription factors,[12] the phosphoinositide-3 kinase (PI3K)/Akt pathway,[13] and the mitogen-activated protein kinase (MAPK) pathway,[14] which promote cell proliferation, differentiation, and survival via multiple effectors.[15] Thus, the *JAK2*V617F mutation constitutively activates JAK2 signaling leading to dysregulated myeloid cell proliferation in most patients with MPNs.[16] Further molecular characterization identified *JAK2* exon 12 mutations in most cases of *JAK2*V617F-negative PV[17] and mutations in the thrombopoietin receptor *MPL*, such as *MPL*W515 L and *MPL*W515 K in *JAK2*V617F-negative patients with ET/MF, accounting for 5% to 10% of ET and MF.[18] As *JAK2*V617F, these mutations induce hyperactive JAK2 signaling and uncontrolled growth of myeloid lineages. Recently, acquired mutations in the chaperone protein calreticulin (*CALR*) were identified in most patients with ET/MF who were *JAK2*-unmutated and *MPL*-unmutated, accounting for 25% to 35% of ET and MF.[19,20] There is mechanistic evidence that *CALR* mutations converge on activation of MPL through facilitating binding of mutant CALR to MPL.[21–24] Thus, mutations in *JAK2, CALR,* and *MPL*, as well as rare mutations in negative regulators of JAK2, such as *LNK* and *CBL*, all induce activated JAK2 signaling. They are mutually exclusive, which highlights the JAK2 pathway activation as a shared mechanism of transformation in MPNs. Transcriptional profiling of MPN granulocytes substantiated this notion, showing gene expression profiles consistent with activated JAK2 signaling in all patients with MPNs independent of mutational status and clinical phenotype.[25] Additional genetic lesions, such as mutations in epigenetic modifiers *TET2, ASXL1, EZH2,* or *IDH1/2,* or in tumor suppressors, such as *TP53*, have also been identified in MPNs and may shape the heterogeneous phenotypes of MPNs and impact the course,[26] whereas JAK-STAT pathway activation represents the central mechanism in the pathogenesis of all MPNs.[25]

The critical role of hyperactive JAK2 signaling in MPN has led to the development of JAK2 inhibitors.[27–31] Conventional JAK2 inhibitors act as ATP mimetics and stabilize JAK2 in the active conformation characterized by paradoxic hyperphosphorylation of the JAK2 activation loop (type I JAK inhibition).[32] They effectively reduce splenomegaly and constitutional symptoms in patients with MPN, which means substantial alleviation of symptom burden.[33,34] A survival advantage has been observed compared with placebo or best available therapy.[35,36] Type I JAK inhibitors are not mutant-selective, meaning that they inhibit both mutant JAK2 as well as activated wild-type JAK2 downstream of mutated *MPL* or *CALR*, providing effective treatment in *JAK2* mutant and *JAK2* wild-type patients with MPN. Ruxolitinib, a JAK1/JAK2 inhibitor has been approved in the United States and Europe for treatment of intermediate-risk and high-risk MF and for PV resistant or intolerant to hydroxyurea. Similar compounds are in clinical development. Momelotinib, a JAK1/JAK2 inhibitor, is currently being compared with ruxolitinib in a phase III study in MF (NCT01969838) and has led to transfusion independence in a significant proportion of patients in a previous phase I/II study.[29] BMS911543 was pursued as a more JAK2-selective inhibitor and completed a phase I/II study (NCT01236352), while additional compounds with JAK2/FLT3 inhibitory profile (fedratinib, pacritinib) did not complete phase III studies due to occurrence of adverse events. Overall, type I JAK2 inhibitors represent a major step forward for the treatment of MPNs, but they have not met the high expectations. A convincing body of evidence demonstrates that they are unable to substantially repress the mutant clone. This inability to induce significant reductions of mutant allele burden suggests a limited curative potential.[2] Moreover, type I JAK inhibitors induce resistance on prolonged exposure, and we also observed cross-resistance among several type I JAK inhibitors in clinical development.[37,38] Given the limited curative potential of type I JAK2 inhibitors, extended duration of treatment is critical to achieve long-term disease control with these agents. Therefore, a detailed understanding of resistance mechanisms is very relevant to inform the development of superior treatment strategies for MPN. Innovative therapeutic approaches to overcome resistance to type I JAK inhibitors are needed.

RESISTANCE TO JAK2 INHIBITORS

Response to type I JAK2 inhibitors can be lost on prolonged exposure, indicating development of resistance in vitro and in vivo. Several mechanisms of resistance to type I JAK2 inhibitors have been identified in MPN cell lines and murine models, including acquired JAK2 kinase mutations,[39,40] persistence of JAK-STAT signaling due to JAK family heterodimer formation,[37,38,41] or protective cytokine effects[42] (**Fig. 1** and **Table 1**). Reports about resistance to type I JAK inhibitor therapy in patients with MPNs are increasing.[43,44]

Molecular Mechanisms of JAK2 Inhibitor Resistance

Genetic resistance

Resistance to tyrosine kinase inhibitors due to acquired mutations is a common theme in therapeutic targeting of oncogenic tyrosine kinases in hematologic malignancies and solid tumors. Mutations usually affect the drug binding site and substantially increase IC_{50} (inhibitory concentration is reduced by half) values as a result of selective pressure on the malignant cell. In chronic myeloid leukemia (CML), an increasing armamentarium of BCR-ABL inhibitors helps to address mutational resistance, whereas resistance mutations are also seen in KIT-driven, platelet-derived growth factor receptor alpha (PDGFRα)-driven, epidermal growth factor receptor (EGFR)-driven and other tyrosine kinase–driven cancers. In MPNs, saturation mutagenesis screens demonstrated the emergence of acquired second-site mutations in *JAK2*, which mediate resistance to type I JAK2 inhibitors. In a *JAK2*V617F expressing cell line, the *JAK2* kinase domain mutations Y931C, G935R, R938L, I960V, and E985K were identified, which are located within and in close proximity to the drug binding pocket.[39] They increased IC_{50} values 9-fold to 33-fold and provided a growth advantage under ruxolitinib. These mutations also conferred cross-resistance to other type I JAK inhibitors in clinical development, such as momelotinib, fedratinib, lestaurtinib, and AZD1480. Mutations at residue M929 corresponding to the gatekeeper mutations

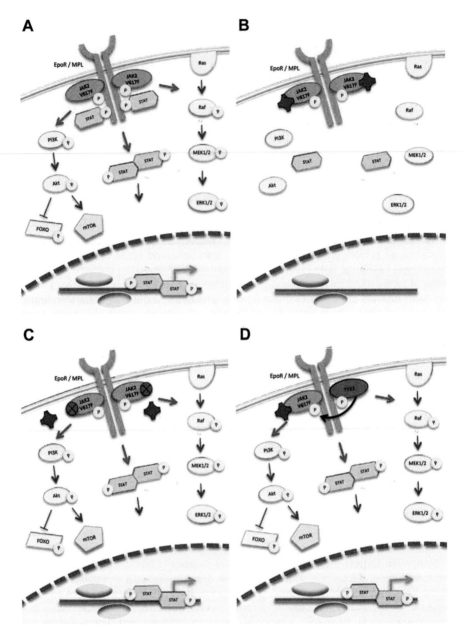

Fig. 1. Mechanisms of resistance to JAK2 inhibitors. (*A*) In MPN, JAK2 signaling is constitutively activated by the acquired *JAK2*V617F mutation in most cases or alternatively by *JAK2* exon 12, *MPL,* or *CALR* mutations (not shown), leading to downstream activation of STAT, PI3K/Akt/mTOR, and MAPK signaling pathways. (*B*) Type I JAK2 inhibitors (shown in *black*) stabilize JAK2 in the active, phosphorylated form and thereby suppress downstream signaling pathways. (*C*) Genetic resistance to type I JAK2 inhibition due to resistance mutations (shown in *red*) is observed in MPN cells in vitro, but has not been reported in patients with MPN so far. (*D*) Resistance to type I JAK2 inhibition in the absence of acquired second-site mutations arises from JAK family heterodimer formation of JAK2 with TYK2 (shown in *purple*) or JAK1 (not shown) and transactivation of JAK2 leading to persistent JAK2 signaling. Further resistance mechanisms include protective cytokine effects and intrinsic resistance in myelofibrosis, which are not depicted and are discussed in the text.

Table 1
Mechanisms of resistance to JAK2 inhibitors in myeloproliferative neoplasms (MPNs)

Resistance	Mechanism	Genetic Alteration	JAK2 Inhibitor	Cross-Resistance	Reversibility	Reference
Genetic resistance	JAK2 mutations	Y931C, G935R, R938L, I960V, E985K	Ruxolitinib	Momelotinib Fedratinib Lestaurtinib AZD1480 Ruxolitinib	No	Deshpande et al,[39] 2012
		Y931C, E864K, G935R	BVB-808	Fedratinib JAK inhibitor I BSK805 tofacitinib	No	Weigert et al,[40] 2012
	Short JAK2 variant	FERM-JAK2	Ruxolitinib	Fedratinib	No	Gorantla et al,[46] 2013
Functional resistance	Persistence of JAK2 signaling based on formation of JAK family heterodimers	None	Ruxolitinib, JAK inhibitor I	Fedratinib	Yes	Koppikar et al,[37] 2012
		None	Ruxolitinib	Ruxolitinib		
			Momelotinib Fedratinib	Momelotinib Fedratinib	Yes	Meyer et al,[38] 2015
			BMS911543	BMS911543		
	Paracrine protective effects by cytokines (interleukin-6, fibroblast growth factor)	n.d.	Atiprimod	n.d.	n.d	Manshouri et al,[42] 2011
	Intrinsic resistance in myelofibrosis	n.d.	Ruxolitinib Momelotinib Lestaurtinib	n.d.	No	Kalota et al,[49] 2013

Several mechanisms of resistance to current JAK2 inhibitors (type I JAK2 inhibitors) have been elucidated including JAK2 resistance mutations, functional adaptation of MPN cells with persistent JAK2 signaling due to JAK family heterodimers, protective cytokine effects, or intrinsic resistance in myelofibrosis. Mutational resistance has not been observed in patients with MPN to date.

Abbreviation: n.d., not done.

T315I in BCR-ABL, T670I in KIT, T674I in PDGFRα, or T790M in EGFR, did not spontaneously occur on inhibitor exposure, and when introduced into *JAK2*, M929I conferred resistance only to ruxolitinib but not to other type I JAK2 inhibitors. A similar screen in cells expressing *JAK2* R683 G, which occurs in CRLF2-rearranged B-cell acute lymphoblastic leukemia (B-ALL), also led to emergence of the Y931C and G935R *JAK2* kinase domain mutations that analogously mediated resistance to multiple type I JAK2 inhibitors in vitro.[40] Acquired mutations of analogous residues in *JAK1* also conferred resistance to ruxolitinib, which mediates its effects via JAK1/JAK2 inhibition.[45] It is important to note that none of these acquired *JAK2* resistance mutations has been reported in patients with MPN to date. Andreoli and colleagues[44] sequenced the *JAK2* kinase domain in 16 of 41 patients with myelofibrosis who developed resistance on ruxolitinib treatment, and did not detect any mutations affecting drug binding. As an additional form of genetic resistance to type I JAK inhibitors, a short *JAK2* variant consisting of kinase and FERM (4.1, ezrin, radixin, moesin (FERM) domain) domains was reported. The JAK2-FERM variant activated STAT5 independently of cytokine receptor binding.[46] However, like acquired *JAK2* kinase mutations, the *JAK2-FERM* variant has not been identified in patients with MPN on JAK inhibitor treatment so far. Mutational resistance to type I JAK inhibitors has exclusively been observed in familial patients with hereditary thrombocytosis based on germline *JAK2* kinase mutations, which were apparently preexisting and not evoked by JAK2 inhibitor treatment.[47] Along with the modest effect of type I JAK2 inhibitors on mutant allele burden in patients with MPN, the absence of acquired resistance mutations provoked by type I JAK2 inhibitors could indicate submaximal target inhibition by these agents without a biological need for genetic escape.

Functional resistance by persistence of JAK-STAT signaling

Beyond genetic adaptation, MPN cells may functionally adapt to JAK2 inhibition causing resistance. Ruxolitinib and other type I JAK inhibitors, such as momelotinib, BMS911543, or fedratinib, stabilize JAK2 in the active conformation and effectively suppress JAK-STAT signaling initially.[32] On prolonged exposure to type I JAK inhibitors, reactivation of JAK-STAT signaling has been observed in *JAK2*V617F and *MPL*W515L mutant MPN cells, which overrides the antiproliferative and apoptosis-inducing effects of type I JAK inhibitors. This functional adaptation is enabled by heterodimer formation of JAK2 with JAK1 or TYK2, which transactivate inhibitor-bound JAK2 and thus enable restoration of downstream signaling.[37] Formation of JAK family heterodimers occurs in *JAK2*-mutant and *MPL*-mutant cell lines and murine models on prolonged exposure to type I JAK inhibitors, and is also seen in patients with MPN on long-term ruxolitinib treatment.

   Of note, resistance to type I JAK inhibitors by JAK family heterodimer formation has been characterized as a reversible process. Withdrawal of the drug restores canonical JAK-STAT signaling as well as responsiveness to type I JAK inhibition.[37] This finding is relevant for the management of ruxolitinib resistance in the clinic and suggests intermittent treatment with type I JAK inhibitors as an option that deserves further evaluation.[43] However, similar to genetic resistance, functional resistance through JAK family heterodimer formation renders MPN cells cross-resistant to several type I JAK inhibitors that are currently in clinical development.[37,38] This could mean that switching treatment from one type I JAK inhibitor to another might not prove as helpful in patients with MPN as in CML, in which in resistance the next line of treatment can be chosen from an array of inhibitors according to mutational profile. The availability of several approved compounds in the near future will help to delineate the exact dynamics of resistance through persistent JAK-STAT signaling on sequential treatment with different type I JAK inhibitors. Furthermore, it is an important observation that MPN cells resistant to type I JAK2 inhibition with ruxolitinib remain JAK2 dependent in vitro and in vivo as shown by knockdown studies.[48] It demonstrates that JAK2 is still a vulnerable target in functionally JAK2 inhibitor–resistant MPN cells. It supports the notion that type I JAK2 inhibition might not be hitting the target effectively enough and encourages the development of more potent classes of JAK2 inhibitors.

Functional resistance by protective cytokine effects

Development of resistance to JAK2 inhibitors also may depend on interactions of the MPN clone with its bone marrow microenvironment. Several cytokines, including interleukin 6 (IL-6) and fibroblast growth factor (FGF), were shown to protect *JAK2*V617F-mutant cells from treatment with a JAK2/JAK3 inhibitor in a paracrine manner.[42] When MPN cell lines or MPN patient mononuclear cells were exposed to stromal cells by in vitro coculture, the suppressing effect of JAK2 inhibition on STAT signaling, proliferation, and survival was reduced. Incubation with stromal cell line supernatant mediated analogous effects, but was ablated on addition of monoclonal antibodies binding the respective cytokines.

Intrinsic resistance in myelofibrosis

Studies on signaling of granulocytes in patients with MPN revealed differential sensitivity of MPN cells to JAK2 inhibition depending on MPN phenotype. STAT5 phosphorylation was less responsive to JAK2 inhibition with lestaurtinib, ruxolitinib, or momelotinib in granulocytes from patients with myelofibrosis than from patients with PV or ET.[49] Patients had no prior JAK inhibitor treatment and this finding was independent of mutant allele burden or cytokine effects. As the causative factors have remained elusive so far, relative resistance of STAT signaling to JAK2 inhibition in MF granulocytes was termed "intrinsic," and further studies are needed to elucidate the functional basis. The findings are relevant regarding the stage of MPN that might benefit most from JAK2 inhibition. Treatment with JAK2 inhibitors in the PV or ET phase could potentially lead to superior therapeutic responses than in progressed post-PV/ET myelofibrosis based on these results, and assessment of prefibrotic versus overt MF also could be worthwhile.

Clinical Aspects of JAK2 Inhibitor Resistance

As JAK2 inhibitor therapy for patients with MPN was introduced into clinical practice relatively recently, characterization of clinical response and resistance to JAK2 inhibitors is not yet as refined as in other tyrosine kinase–driven malignancies, such as for example, CML. Some studies consider *primary resistance* to JAK2 inhibitors as absent or minor reduction of splenomegaly and constitutional symptoms and *secondary resistance* as a recurrence of splenomegaly and constitutional symptoms after initial response.[44] As most patients with MPN promptly respond to ruxolitinib, loss of response and consecutive discontinuation of treatment prevail. Andreoli and colleagues[44] reported ruxolitinib resistance in 41% of patients with myelofibrosis mostly after extended exposure of more than 1 year. Resistance was characterized by renewed splenomegaly, whereas half of the patients also suffered from recurrent constitutional symptoms. No resistance mutations in the *JAK2* kinase domain were detected. Resistance to ruxolitinib was more frequently seen in patients with high-risk disease according to International Prognostic Scoring System (IPSS) score and was associated with the absence of *JAK2, MPL, TET2,* and *SRSF2* mutations, whereas *CALR* mutations were not evaluated. A recent analysis by Patel and colleagues[50] found poor spleen response to ruxolitinib and shorter time to treatment discontinuation significantly enriched in patients with 1 or more mutations in *ASXL1*, *EZH2*, or *IDH1/2*, which were previously related to adverse outcome.[26] Presence of 3 or more mutations from a 28-gene panel, including known driver mutations as well as mutations associated with disease initiation and progression in MPN predicted suboptimal efficacy of ruxolitinib treatment, as well as shorter overall survival. Taken together, these studies suggest that ruxolitinib resistance preferentially occurs in patients with high-risk myelofibrosis as judged by IPSS score and mutational profile. Concordant with in vitro studies on adaptive resistance in the absence of resistance mutations, ruxolitinib resistance was reversible after withdrawal of the drug, even if paused for only a couple of days.[43] Resumption of treatment achieved renewed response of splenomegaly and constitutional symptoms, although for a shorter period or to a lesser extent than with first exposure.

APPROACHES TO OVERCOME RESISTANCE TO JAK2 INHIBITORS IN MYELOPROLIFERATIVE NEOPLASMS

Malignant cells driven by constitutively active tyrosine kinases inevitably find ways to develop resistance to tyrosine kinase inhibitors, as observed in hematological and solid cancers including MPN. Novel therapeutic approaches that hold promise for overcoming resistance to current JAK2 inhibitors in MPN, are at different stages of development (**Table 2**).

Type I JAK2 Inhibitors

First reports suggest that pausing ruxolitinib therapy reverses resistance in patients with MPN and may lead to renewed sensitivity thereafter for shorter periods.[43] A phase II study on retreatment of patients with myelofibrosis with ruxolitinib after treatment interruption due to loss of response aimed to assess efficacy and safety of restarting ruxolitinib, but was terminated due to low enrollment (ReTreatment Trial, NCT02091752). It will be important to carefully evaluate safety and toxicity aspects of this strategy, as pausing ruxolitinib may cause flaring of symptoms due to a rebound of cytokines. To avoid development of resistance to type I JAK2 inhibitors, alternative dosing regimens, such as intermittent treatment with higher-dose pulses, have been proposed.[51] Besides ruxolitinib, additional type I JAK2 inhibitors are currently in clinical trials, such as momelotinib, which is being compared with ruxolitinib in a head-to-head phase III study (NCT01969838) and is also evaluated for duration of splenic response in long-term follow-up (NCT02124746). Experience on the potential of momelotinib or other type I JAK inhibitors on ruxolitinib resistance is still limited and will accumulate after approval and broader use of these compounds. Given the in vitro data on type I JAK inhibitor cross-resistance,[37–40] cross-resistance of type I JAK2 inhibitors should be considered a possible scenario also in clinical application. Unlike reports of genetic cross-resistance to ruxolitinib and fedratinib,[39] a recent study described absence of resistance mutations to fedratinib due to its ability to bind both the ATP-binding and the substrate-binding site of JAK2.[52]

That treatment by current type I JAK2 inhibitors does not evoke resistance mutations in patients with MPN and the finding that type I JAK2 inhibitor–resistant MPN cells remain dependent on JAK2 signaling,[48] suggest incomplete target inhibition. It calls for more thorough suppression of JAK2 signaling in treatment-naïve and treatment-resistant patients with MPN. This may occur by more potent targeting of JAK2 itself or by additional targeting of factors contributing to the oncogenic signal downstream of activated JAK2. Several approaches are being studied.

Table 2
Approaches to overcome JAK2 inhibitor resistance in myeloproliferative neoplasms (MPNs)

Class	Concept	Agent	Evidence for Resolution of Resistance				Reference
			MPN Cells	Murine Models	Patient Samples	Patients/Clinical Trials	
Type I JAK2 inhibitors	Intermittent administration	Ruxolitinib	+	n.d.	n.d.	NCT02091752 (terminated)	Gisslinger et al,[43] 2014; Shank et al,[51] 2014
	Targeting substrate-binding site	Fedratinib	+	n.d.	n.d.	n.d.	Kesarwani et al,[52] 2015
HSP90 inhibitors	Targeting chaperone function to reduce JAK2 levels	PU-H71	+	+	+	NCT01393509	Marubayashi et al,[53] 2010; Koppikar et al,[37] 2012; Bhagwat et al,[48] 2014
		AUY922	+	+	n.d.	NCT01668173 (terminated)	Weigert et al,[40] 2012
Type II JAK2 inhibition	Targeting inactive conformation of JAK2	BBT594	+	n.d.	n.d.	n.d.	Andraos et al,[32] 201; Koppikar et al,[37] 2012
		CH2868	+	+	+	n.d.	Meyer et al,[38] 2015
PI3K/Akt/mTOR inhibition	Targeting additional signaling pathways combined with type I JAK2 inhibition	MK-2206 BEZ235	+	+	+	n.d.	Khan et al,[55] 2013; Fiskus et al,[57] 2013
PI3K/Akt + MEK inhibition		MK-2206 + AZD6244	+	n.d.	n.d.	n.d.	Winter et al,[59] 2014
PIM kinase inhibition		AZD1208	+	n.d.	+	n.d.	Huang et al,[60] 2014; Mazzacurati et al,[61] 2015
Bcl-2/Bcl-xL inhibition		ABT737	+	+	n.d.	n.d.	Waibel et al,[41] 2013

Intermittent administration of type I JAK2 inhibitors, more effective targeting of JAK2 by HSP90 inhibition or type II JAK2 inhibition as well as combination therapy approaches are being studied to provide therapeutic approaches overcoming JAK2 inhibitor resistance in MPN.
Abbreviations: +, Yes; mTOR, mammalian target of rapamycin; n.d., not done.

Heat Shock Protein 90 Inhibition

Heat shock protein 90 (HSP90) represents a chaperone protein involved in posttranscriptional stabilization and conformational maturation of multiple client proteins, including oncogenic factors implicated in the growth and survival of malignant cells. JAK2 has been identified as an HSP90 client and is susceptible to HSP90 inhibition.[53] In MPN cell lines, murine models and ex vivo treated patient samples, HSP90 inhibition reduced phosphorylated and total JAK2 expression and decreased downstream signaling activity. The finding of decreased JAK2 total protein levels on HSP90 inhibition is meaningful, as knockdown of JAK2 has shown major corrective effects in MPN cells resistant to JAK2 inhibitors.[48] HSP90 inhibitors, including PU-H71 and AUY922, retained activity in MPN cells in vitro, in vivo, or in patient samples. In *MPL*W515L or *Jak2*V617F mutated mouse models pretreated with ruxolitinib, combined Jak2 and HSP90 inhibition provided further improved results, including reduction of mutant allele burden. These favorable results pose HSP90 inhibition with PU-H71 and AUY922 as a valid approach to abrogate type I JAK2 inhibitor resistance.[37,40,48] An open-label phase II study of AUY922 yielded promising results in patients with myelofibrosis and PV/ET refractory to conventional therapy, but was terminated due to occurrence of gastrointestinal adverse events (NCT01668173). PU-H71 is being evaluated in a first-in-human phase I trial in patients with MPN with previous ruxolitinib therapy and persistent disease manifestations, which will inform us about the potential of HSP90 inhibition in JAK2 inhibitor resistance (NCT01393509). Thus, HSP90 inhibition provides a promising approach for more effective targeting of JAK2 in treatment-naïve and in type I JAK2 inhibitor–resistant patients with MPN. Concerns that HSP90 inhibition could interfere with the functions of other HSP90 client proteins should prompt close evaluation of toxicities.

Type II JAK2 Inhibition

In contrast to type I JAK2 inhibitors, which stabilize the active conformation of JAK2, type II JAK2 inhibitors block JAK2 enzymatic activity in the inactive conformation. They bind a hydrophobic site adjacent to the ATP-binding pocket uncovered in the inactive conformation of JAK2 in which the activation loop is in the "DFG motif-out" state with phenylalanine F995 of the activation loop dislocated by 10 Å.[32] This alternative mode of JAK2 inhibition gained important interest due to the limitations of type I JAK2 inhibitors and as type II inhibition is successfully used for targeting of other tyrosine kinases, such as BCR-ABL. The first type II inhibitor reported for JAK2, BBT594, was designed for targeting of T315I mutated BCR-ABL, but revealed activity against JAK2.[32] BBT594 remains active in type I JAK2 inhibitor–resistant cells,[37] but is limited to in vitro application. Drug discovery efforts led to the development of CHZ868, a type II JAK2 inhibitor with an optimized profile. CHZ868 is highly active in MPN[38] and in JAK2-driven ALL[54] in vitro and in vivo, reducing proliferation and inducing apoptosis in malignant cells. It retains activity in type I JAK2 inhibitor–resistant MPN cells effectively suppressing proliferation and inducing apoptosis, and it abrogates the persistent signaling in MPN patient samples after long-term ruxolitinib treatment. Type II JAK2 inhibition by CHZ868 inhibits both mutant and wild-type JAK2, but in contrast to type I JAK2 inhibition, hematopoietic cells expressing Jak2V617F show higher sensitivity to the antiproliferative effect of CHZ868 versus cells with wild-type Jak2. In MPN models in vivo, the mutant compartment showed increased susceptibility to apoptosis induction by CHZ868. Thus, CHZ868 is able to effectively reduce mutant allele burden in several MPN mouse models,[38] and similar findings were reported for JAK2-driven ALL,[54] which suggests type II JAK2 inhibition as an option for development of more mutant-targeted clinical JAK2 inhibitors., Hematologic toxicities are not increased on type II JAK2 inhibition.[54] Thus, the alternative mode of type II JAK2 inhibition holds promise for the management of resistance to the conventional type I JAK2 inhibitors, such as ruxolitinib, as well as for the development of JAK2 inhibitors with disease-modifying potential. The preferential targeting of the mutant MPN clone seen with type II JAK2 inhibition is meaningful, as truly mutant-selective JAK2 inhibitors have not yet been reported.

Combination Therapy Approaches

The signaling network downstream of activated JAK2, including PI3K/Akt/mTOR and MAPK pathways, PIM kinases, or the Bcl-2/Bcl-xL family of apoptosis regulators, represent additional targets in MPN, and their inhibition could contribute to abrogation of JAK2 inhibitor resistance. Recurrent mutations in epigenetic modifiers, such as TET2, IDH1/2, ASXL1, and EZH2, in MPN suggested interference with chromatin modification as a promising therapeutic concept. Based on these molecular insights, multiple combination therapy approaches with JAK2 inhibitors are in development and some are specifically evaluated for efficacy in JAK2 inhibitor resistance.

PI3K/Akt/Mammalian Target of Rapamycin Pathway

The PI3K/Akt/mammalian target of rapamycin (mTOR) pathway has been targeted by several agents in combination with JAK2 inhibition. The Akt inhibitor MK-2206 was effective in MPN cells and murine models synergistically with ruxolitinib,[55] whereas the mTOR inhibitor everolimus showed activity in a phase I/II study in myelofibrosis.[56] The dual PI3K/mTOR inhibitor BEZ235 was remarkable, as BEZ235 was shown to overcome resistance to type I JAK2 inhibitor resistance in MPN cells.[57] Based on the activation of the MAPK signaling pathway in MPN, combined JAK2 and Akt inhibition plus MEK inhibition was also effective.[58,59]

PIM Kinases

PIM kinases have recently been recognized as a promising therapeutic target in MPN induced by JAK-STAT signaling. PIMs promote survival of MPN cells via multiple factors, including MYC, which was indicated as central target by short hairpin RNA screens for combination therapies.[60] Combined pan-PIM and JAK2 inhibition with ruxolitinib or TG101348 synergistically reduced proliferation and induced apoptosis of MPN cells. Importantly, PIM/JAK2 inhibitor combinations were effective in type I JAK2 inhibitor–resistant MPN cells and further studies are awaited to validate combined PIM/JAK2 inhibition as an approach to overcome JAK2 inhibitor resistance.[60,61]

Bcl-2/Bcl-xL Inhibition

Bcl-2/Bcl-xL inhibition in combination with JAK2 inhibition has attracted interest, as prosurvival Bcl-2 family genes were shown to be upregulated in JAK2-driven hematological malignancies, including JAK2V617F-mutant MPN, JAK2R683G-mutant B-ALL, and TEL-JAK rearranged T-ALL. Combined targeting of Bcl-2/Bcl-xL and JAK2 by the Bcl-2/Bcl-xL inhibitor, ABT737 and ruxolitinib significantly prolonged survival in respective mouse models.[41] Of note, combined Bcl-2/Bcl-xL and JAK2 inhibitor treatment could prevent development of JAK2 inhibitor resistance or overcome established resistance in JAK2V617F-mutant MPN cells by interference with these prosurvival apoptosis regulators.

Pan-Histone Deacetylase Inhibitors

Pan-histone deacetylase (HDAC) inhibitors, such as panobinostat, are promising compounds for MPN therapy known to enhance histone H3 and H4 acetylation and inhibiting HSP90 chaperone function.[62] Panobinostat effectively interfered with expression, activation, and downstream signaling of JAK2 and showed activity in a phase I study in myelofibrosis.[63] Combination therapy with type I JAK2 inhibition by TG101348[62] or ruxolitinib[64] showed superior effects in *JAK2*V617F MPN cells and murine models, which led to ongoing phase I trials (NCT01433445, NCT01693601). However, the specific potential of panobinostat to overcome type I JAK2 inhibitor resistance has not been evaluated so far.

Additional Novel Concepts

Additional novel concepts of MPN therapy are currently emerging. Targeting telomerase enzymatic activity by inhibition of human telomerase reverse transcriptase has proven efficacious in phase I/II studies of imetelstat in MF[65] and ET,[66] but myelosuppressive effects need to be considered (NCT01731951, NCT01243073). Based on the observation that sympathetic neural signals and consecutively nestin$^+$ mesenchymal stem cells are reduced in the MPN bone marrow niche, sympathomimetic agents were administered in *JAK2*V617F murine models and blocked MPN progression.[67] A phase II efficacy study with the sympathomimetic agonist mirabegron is currently in progress in *JAK2*V617F-mutant PV, ET, and MF (NCT02311569). In addition, dysregulated megakaryopoiesis, which represents a hallmark in MPN pathogenesis and promotes bone marrow fibrosis, was successfully targeted by inhibition of Aurora kinases in murine models of MF,[68] while fresolimumab, a monoclonal antibody against transforming growth factor (TGF)-β is under evaluation in a phase I study (NCT01291784) based on the role of TGF-β in promoting fibrosis. All these approaches are based on the increasing insight into the molecular processes contributing to MPN development. With regard to their future application in MPN therapy, it will be of major interest to test their potential to overcome resistance to type I JAK2 inhibitors as a next step.

Type I JAK2 inhibition has substantially advanced MPN therapy by initiating the era of molecularly targeting the JAK2 tyrosine kinase as the main pathogenic driver. Current efforts for a detailed understanding of the limitations including mechanisms of type I JAK2 inhibitor resistance are well invested. They will prove rewarding by informing the development of next-stage targeted agents and combinatorial treatment concepts that will override JAK2 inhibitor resistance and will advance our therapeutic options for patients with MPN.

REFERENCES

1. Titmarsh GJ, Duncombe AS, McMullin MF, et al. How common are myeloproliferative neoplasms? A systematic review and meta-analysis. Am J Hematol 2014; 89(6):581–7.

2. Mughal TI, Barbui T, Abdel-Wahab O, et al. Novel insights into the biology and treatment of chronic myeloproliferative neoplasms. Leuk Lymphoma 2015;56(7): 1938–48.

3. Tefferi A, Vaidya R, Caramazza D, et al. Circulating interleukin (IL)-8, IL-2R, IL-12, and IL-15 levels are independently prognostic in primary myelofibrosis: a comprehensive cytokine profiling study. J Clin Oncol 2011;29(10):1356–63.

4. Gangat N, Caramazza D, Vaidya R, et al. DIPSS plus: a refined Dynamic International Prognostic Scoring System for primary myelofibrosis that incorporates

prognostic information from karyotype, platelet count, and transfusion status. J Clin Oncol 2011;29(4):392–7.

5. Levine RL, Wadleigh M, Cools J, et al. Activating mutation in the tyrosine kinase JAK2 in polycythemia vera, essential thrombocythemia, and myeloid metaplasia with myelofibrosis. Cancer cell 2005;7(4):387–97.

6. Kralovics R, Passamonti F, Buser AS, et al. A gain-of-function mutation of JAK2 in myeloproliferative disorders. N Engl J Med 2005;352(17):1779–90.

7. Baxter EJ, Scott LM, Campbell PJ, et al. Acquired mutation of the tyrosine kinase JAK2 in human myeloproliferative disorders. Lancet 2005;365(9464):1054–61.

8. James C, Ugo V, Le Couedic JP, et al. A unique clonal JAK2 mutation leading to constitutive signalling causes polycythaemia vera. Nature 2005;434(7037):1144–8.

9. Neubauer H, Cumano A, Muller M, et al. Jak2 deficiency defines an essential developmental checkpoint in definitive hematopoiesis. Cell 1998;93(3):397–409.

10. Parganas E, Wang D, Stravopodis D, et al. Jak2 is essential for signaling through a variety of cytokine receptors. Cell 1998;93(3):385–95.

11. Lu X, Levine R, Tong W, et al. Expression of a homodimeric type I cytokine receptor is required for JAK2V617F-mediated transformation. Proc Natl Acad Sci U S A 2005;102(52):18962–7.

12. Walz C, Ahmed W, Lazarides K, et al. Essential role for Stat5a/b in myeloproliferative neoplasms induced by BCR-ABL1 and JAK2(V617F) in mice. Blood 2012;119(15):3550–60.

13. Kamishimoto J, Tago K, Kasahara T, et al. Akt activation through the phosphorylation of erythropoietin receptor at tyrosine 479 is required for myeloproliferative disorder-associated JAK2 V617F mutant-induced cellular transformation. Cell Signal 2011;23(5):849–56.

14. Wolf A, Eulenfeld R, Gabler K, et al. JAK2-V617F-induced MAPK activity is regulated by PI3K and acts synergistically with PI3K on the proliferation of JAK2-V617F-positive cells. JAKSTAT 2013;2(3):e24574.

15. Skoda RC, Duek A, Grisouard J. Pathogenesis of myeloproliferative neoplasms. Exp Hematol 2015;43(8):599–608.

16. Silvennoinen O, Hubbard SR. Molecular insights into regulation of JAK2 in myeloproliferative neoplasms. Blood 2015;125(22):3388–92.

17. Scott LM, Tong W, Levine RL, et al. JAK2 exon 12 mutations in polycythemia vera and idiopathic erythrocytosis. N Engl J Med 2007;356(5):459–68.

18. Pikman Y, Lee BH, Mercher T, et al. MPLW515L is a novel somatic activating mutation in myelofibrosis with myeloid metaplasia. PLoS Med 2006;3(7):e270.

19. Klampfl T, Gisslinger H, Harutyunyan AS, et al. Somatic mutations of calreticulin in myeloproliferative neoplasms. N Engl J Med 2013;369(25):2379–90.

20. Nangalia J, Massie CE, Baxter EJ, et al. Somatic CALR mutations in myeloproliferative neoplasms with nonmutated JAK2. N Engl J Med 2013;369(25):2391–405.

21. Elf S, Abdelfattah NS, Chen E, et al. Mutant calreticulin requires both its mutant C-terminus and the thrombopoietin receptor for oncogenic transformation. Cancer Discov 2016;6(4):368–81.

22. Araki M, Yang Y, Masubuchi N, et al. Activation of the thrombopoietin receptor by mutant calreticulin in CALR-mutant myeloproliferative neoplasms. Blood 2016;127(10):1307–16.

23. Marty C, Pecquet C, Nivarthi H, et al. Calreticulin mutants in mice induce an MPL-dependent thrombocytosis with frequent progression to myelofibrosis. Blood 2015;127(10):1317–24.

24. Chachoua I, Pecquet C, El-Khoury M, et al. Thrombopoietin receptor activation by myeloproliferative neoplasm associated calreticulin mutants. Blood 2016; 127(10):1325–35.

25. Rampal R, Al-Shahrour F, Abdel-Wahab O, et al. Integrated genomic analysis illustrates the central role of JAK-STAT pathway activation in myeloproliferative neoplasm pathogenesis. Blood 2014;123(22):e123–33.

26. Tefferi A, Abdel-Wahab O, Cervantes F, et al. Mutations with epigenetic effects in myeloproliferative neoplasms and recent progress in treatment: Proceedings from the 5th International Post-ASH Symposium. Blood Cancer J 2011;1:e7.

27. Verstovsek S, Kantarjian H, Mesa RA, et al. Safety and efficacy of INCB018424, a JAK1 and JAK2 inhibitor, in myelofibrosis. N Engl J Med 2010;363(12):1117–27.

28. Pardanani A, Gotlib JR, Jamieson C, et al. Safety and efficacy of TG101348, a selective JAK2 inhibitor, in myelofibrosis. J Clin Oncol 2011;29(7):789–96.

29. Pardanani A, Laborde RR, Lasho TL, et al. Safety and efficacy of CYT387, a JAK1 and JAK2 inhibitor, in myelofibrosis. Leukemia 2013;27(6):1322–7.

30. Meyer SC, Levine RL. Molecular pathways: molecular basis for sensitivity and resistance to JAK kinase inhibitors. Clin Cancer Res 2014;20(8):2051–9.

31. Verstovsek SO, Scott O, Estrov B, et al. Phase I dose-escalation trial of SB1518, a novel JAK2/FLT3 inhibitor, in acute and chronic myeloid diseases, including primary or post-essential thrombocythemia/polycythemia vera myelofibrosis. Blood 2009;114:3905.

32. Andraos R, Qian Z, Bonenfant D, et al. Modulation of activation-loop phosphorylation by JAK inhibitors is binding mode dependent. Cancer Discov 2012;2(6): 512–23.

33. Verstovsek S, Mesa RA, Gotlib J, et al. A double-blind, placebo-controlled trial of ruxolitinib for myelofibrosis. N Engl J Med 2012;366(9):799–807.

34. Harrison C, Kiladjian JJ, Al-Ali HK, et al. JAK inhibition with ruxolitinib versus best available therapy for myelofibrosis. N Engl J Med 2012;366(9):787–98.

35. Verstovsek S, Mesa RA, Gotlib J, et al. Efficacy, safety and survival with ruxolitinib in patients with myelofibrosis: results of a median 2-year follow-up of COMFORT-I. Haematologica 2013;98(12):1865–71.

36. Cervantes F, Vannucchi AM, Kiladjian JJ, et al. Three-year efficacy, safety, and survival findings from COMFORT-II, a phase 3 study comparing ruxolitinib with best available therapy for myelofibrosis. Blood 2013;122(25):4047–53.

37. Koppikar P, Bhagwat N, Kilpivaara O, et al. Heterodimeric JAK-STAT activation as a mechanism of persistence to JAK2 inhibitor therapy. Nature 2012;489(7414): 155–9.

38. Meyer SC, Keller MD, Chiu S, et al. CHZ868, a Type II JAK2 inhibitor, reverses Type I JAK inhibitor persistence and demonstrates efficacy in myeloproliferative neoplasms. Cancer cell 2015;28(1):15–28.

39. Deshpande A, Reddy MM, Schade GO, et al. Kinase domain mutations confer resistance to novel inhibitors targeting JAK2V617F in myeloproliferative neoplasms. Leukemia 2012;26(4):708–15.

40. Weigert O, Lane AA, Bird L, et al. Genetic resistance to JAK2 enzymatic inhibitors is overcome by HSP90 inhibition. J Exp Med 2012;209(2):259–73.

41. Waibel M, Solomon VS, Knight DA, et al. Combined targeting of JAK2 and Bcl-2/Bcl-xL to cure mutant JAK2-driven malignancies and overcome acquired resistance to JAK2 inhibitors. Cell Rep 2013;5(4):1047–59.

42. Manshouri T, Estrov Z, Quintas-Cardama A, et al. Bone marrow stroma-secreted cytokines protect JAK2(V617F)-mutated cells from the effects of a JAK2 inhibitor. Cancer Res 2011;71(11):3831–40.

43. Gisslinger H, Schalling M, Gisslinger B, et al. Restoration of response to ruxolitinib upon brief withdrawal in two patients with myelofibrosis. Am J Hematol 2014; 89(3):344–6.

44. Andreoli AVE, Robin M, Raffoux E, et al. Clinical resistance to ruxolitinib is more frequent in patients without MPN-associated mutations and is rarely due to mutations in the JAK2 kinase drug-binding domain. Blood 2013;(122):1591.

45. Hornakova T, Springuel L, Devreux J, et al. Oncogenic JAK1 and JAK2-activating mutations resistant to ATP-competitive inhibitors. Haematologica 2011;96(6): 845–53.

46. Gorantla SP, Rudelius M, Albers C, et al. Identification of a novel mode of kinase inhibitor resistance in JAK2: JAK2 inhibitor resistance is mediated by the generation of 45-kDa JAK2 variant which alters the kinase domain structure. Blood 2013;(122):113.

47. Marty C, Saint-Martin C, Pecquet C, et al. Germ-line JAK2 mutations in the kinase domain are responsible for hereditary thrombocytosis and are resistant to JAK2 and HSP90 inhibitors. Blood 2014;123(9):1372–83.

48. Bhagwat N, Koppikar P, Keller M, et al. Improved targeting of JAK2 leads to increased therapeutic efficacy in myeloproliferative neoplasms. Blood 2014; 123(13):2075–83.

49. Kalota A, Jeschke GR, Carroll M, et al. Intrinsic resistance to JAK2 inhibition in myelofibrosis. Clin Cancer Res 2013;19(7):1729–39.

50. Patel KP, Newberry KJ, Luthra R, et al. Correlation of mutation profile and response in patients with myelofibrosis treated with ruxolitinib. Blood 2015; 126(6):790–7.

51. Shank K, Bhagwat N, Keller MD, et al. Mathematical optimization of JAK inhibitor dose and scheduling for MPN patients. Blood 2014;(124):911.

52. Kesarwani M, Huber E, Kincaid Z, et al. Targeting substrate-site in Jak2 kinase prevents emergence of genetic resistance. Sci Rep 2015;5:14538.

53. Marubayashi S, Koppikar P, Taldone T, et al. HSP90 is a therapeutic target in JAK2-dependent myeloproliferative neoplasms in mice and humans. J Clin Invest 2010;120(10):3578–93.

54. Wu SC, Li LS, Kopp N, et al. Activity of the type II JAK2 inhibitor CHZ868 in B cell acute lymphoblastic leukemia. Cancer cell 2015;28(1):29–41.

55. Khan I, Huang Z, Wen Q, et al. AKT is a therapeutic target in myeloproliferative neoplasms. Leukemia 2013;27(9):1882–90.

56. Guglielmelli P, Barosi G, Rambaldi A, et al. Safety and efficacy of everolimus, a mTOR inhibitor, as single agent in a phase 1/2 study in patients with myelofibrosis. Blood 2011;118(8):2069–76.

57. Fiskus W, Verstovsek S, Manshouri T, et al. Dual PI3K/AKT/mTOR inhibitor BEZ235 synergistically enhances the activity of JAK2 inhibitor against cultured and primary human myeloproliferative neoplasm cells. Mol Cancer Ther 2013; 12(5):577–88.

58. Fiskus WMR, Balusu R, Bhalla KN. Synergistic activity of combinations of JAK2 kinase inhibitor with PI3K/mTOR, MEK or PIM kinase inhibitor against human myeloproliferative neoplasm cells expressing JAK2V617F. Blood 2010;(116):798.

59. Winter PS, Sarosiek KA, Lin KH, et al. RAS signaling promotes resistance to JAK inhibitors by suppressing BAD-mediated apoptosis. Sci Signal 2014;7(357): ra122.

60. Huang SM, Wang A, Greco R, et al. Combination of PIM and JAK2 inhibitors synergistically suppresses MPN cell proliferation and overcomes drug resistance. Oncotarget 2014;5(10):3362–74.

61. Mazzacurati L, Lambert QT, Pradhan A, et al. The PIM inhibitor AZD1208 synergizes with ruxolitinib to induce apoptosis of ruxolitinib sensitive and resistant JAK2-V617F-driven cells and inhibit colony formation of primary MPN cells. Oncotarget 2015;6(37):40141–57.

62. Wang Y, Fiskus W, Chong DG, et al. Cotreatment with panobinostat and JAK2 inhibitor TG101209 attenuates JAK2V617F levels and signaling and exerts synergistic cytotoxic effects against human myeloproliferative neoplastic cells. Blood 2009;114(24):5024–33.

63. Mascarenhas J, Lu M, Li T, et al. A phase I study of panobinostat (LBH589) in patients with primary myelofibrosis (PMF) and post-polycythaemia vera/essential thrombocythaemia myelofibrosis (post-PV/ET MF). Br J Haematol 2013;161(1): 68–75.

64. Evrot E, Ebel N, Romanet V, et al. JAK1/2 and Pan-deacetylase inhibitor combination therapy yields improved efficacy in preclinical mouse models of JAK2V617F-driven disease. Clin Cancer Res 2013;19(22):6230–41.

65. Tefferi A, Lasho TL, Begna KH, et al. A pilot study of the telomerase inhibitor imetelstat for myelofibrosis. N Engl J Med 2015;373(10):908–19.

66. Baerlocher GM, Oppliger Leibundgut E, Ottmann OG, et al. Telomerase inhibitor imetelstat in patients with essential thrombocythemia. N Engl J Med 2015; 373(10):920–8.

67. Arranz L, Sanchez-Aguilera A, Martin-Perez D, et al. Neuropathy of haematopoietic stem cell niche is essential for myeloproliferative neoplasms. Nature 2014;512(7512):78–81.

68. Wen QJ, Yang Q, Goldenson B, et al. Targeting megakaryocytic-induced fibrosis in myeloproliferative neoplasms by AURKA inhibition. Nat Med 2015;21(12): 1473–80.

Tyrosine Kinase Inhibitors in the Treatment of Eosinophilic Neoplasms and Systemic Mastocytosis

 CrossMark

Jason Gotlib, MD, MS

KEYWORDS

- Systemic mastocytosis • Hypereosinophilic syndrome • Tyrosine kinase inhibitor
- *FIP1L1-PDGFRA* • *FGFR1* • *JAK2* • Imatinib • Midostaurin

KEY POINTS

- Evaluation of eosinophilia-associated neoplasms and systemic mastocytosis requires diagnostic testing for rearrangements or point mutations involving tyrosine kinase genes.
- Imatinib is a highly effective, first-line therapy for myeloid/lymphoid neoplasms with eosinophilia characterized by *PDGFRA* or *PDGFRB* gene fusions.
- An unmet need exists for treatment of *FGFR1*-rearranged and *JAK2*-rearranged eosinophilic myeloid/lymphoid neoplasms in which currently available tyrosine kinase inhibitors demonstrate suboptimal efficacy.
- Novel agents with potent inhibitory activity against KIT D816V have demonstrated significant clinical benefit and reductions of bone marrow mast cell burden in patients with advanced systemic mastocytosis.

INTRODUCTION

Constitutive activation of tyrosine kinases (TKs) is a common theme among myeloproliferative neoplasms (MPNs), and typically occurs via point mutations or rearrangements. Well-known examples include *BCR-ABL1*, which operationally defines chronic myeloid leukemia (CML), and Janus kinase 2 (*JAK2*) V617F, which is a highly recurrent mutation among the classic Philadelphia chromosome–negative MPNs polycythemia vera, essential thrombocythemia, and primary myelofibrosis.[1] Among the primary (clonal)

Disclosure Statement: Dr J. Gotlib is the Chair of the Study Steering Committee for global trial of midostaurin in advanced systemic mastocytosis, sponsored by Novartis. He has received trial funding from Novartis and Blueprint Medicines, and honoraria for serving on Advisory Boards for Novartis and Deciphera. Dr J. Gotlib also receives reimbursement for travel expenses from Novartis.

Division of Hematology, Stanford Cancer Institute/Stanford University School of Medicine, 875 Blake Wilbur Drive, Room 2324, Stanford, CA 94305-5821, USA
E-mail address: jason.gotlib@stanford.edu

Hematol Oncol Clin N Am 31 (2017) 643–661
http://dx.doi.org/10.1016/j.hoc.2017.04.009
hemonc.theclinics.com

eosinophilias, a subset of patients belongs to the 2016 World Health Organization (WHO) category entitled, "Myeloid/lymphoid neoplasms with eosinophilia and rearrangement of *PDGFRA*, *PDGFRB*, or *FGFR1*, or with *PCM1-JAK2*."[1] In addition to these TK genes, eosinophilic neoplasms may rarely be associated with rearrangement of FMS-like tyrosine kinase 3 (*FLT3*) and *ABL1* (**Table 1**). In systemic mastocytosis (SM), the aspartate to valine mutation in codon 816 (D816 V) in the gene encoding the KIT receptor tyrosine kinase can be identified in approximately 80% to 90% of patients and is a primary driver of disease pathogenesis.[1,2]

Although imatinib treatment of *FIP1L1-PDGFRA*–positive (and *PDGFRB*-rearranged) myeloid neoplasms with eosinophilia has recapitulated the success observed in CML, therapy of other eosinophilic diseases has been more challenging due to the limited potency and selectivity of current of TK inhibitors (TKIs) and disease heterogeneity (**Table 2**). Recently, agents such as midostaurin, a multikinase/KIT inhibitor, have demonstrated encouraging efficacy in patients with advanced SM.[3] In this article, I review the current landscape and challenges of TKI therapy in eosinophilic neoplasms and advanced mast cell disease, and discuss emerging opportunities for progress.

EOSINOPHILIC NEOPLASMS
Imatinib in Patients with PDGFRA/B Fusion Genes

Imatinib's profound benefits in CML led to its empiric use in patients with hypereosinophilia who exhibited myeloproliferative features. In 2001 to 2002, several reports highlighted rapid and complete hematologic responses with imatinib 100 to 400 mg daily in patients with hypereosinophilic syndrome.[4–6] The fusion oncoprotein FIP1L1-PDGFRα, generated by a cytogenetically occult 800-kilobase interstitial deletion on chromosome 4q12, was identified as the target of imatinib.[7,8] The deleted segment contains the *CHIC2* gene, which is the basis for the fluorescence in situ hybridization (FISH) test used to diagnose of *FIP1L1-PDGFRA* disease[9]; FISH and reverse-transcriptase polymerase chain reaction (PCR) can be used for diagnosis, and both assays have been used to monitor cytogenetic and molecular response to imatinib (see **Table 1**). Although *FIP1L1-PDGFRA*–positive disease usually presents as a chronic myeloid neoplasm with eosinophilia, it may be diagnosed in the blastic phase of an MPN, or as an eosinophilia-associated acute myeloid leukemia (AML) or T-cell lymphoblastic lymphoma.[10]

The durable hematologic and molecular remissions induced by imatinib in *FIP1L1-PDGFRA*–positive myeloid neoplasms have been corroborated by many studies (see **Table 2**).[7,11–16] Molecular remissions were first reported by the National Institutes of Health group in 5 of 6 *FIP1L1-PDGFRA*–positive patients after 1 to 12 months of imatinib therapy.[13] Although 100 mg daily may be sufficient to achieve a molecular remission in many patients, others may require higher maintenance doses in the range of 300 to 400 mg daily. Dosing of 100 to 200 mg weekly may be sufficient to maintain long-term molecular remissions in some patients.[17] In a French Eosinophil Network series, a complete hematologic response was achieved in all patients, and complete molecular response (CMR) in 95% of patients (average starting imatinib dose, 165 mg/d).[16]

The disease course of imatinib-treated *FIP1L1-PDGFRA*–positive myeloid neoplasms was studied in a prospective Italian cohort of 27 patients with a median follow-up period of 25 months (range 15–60 months).[12] Patients were dose escalated from an initial dose of 100 mg daily to a final dose of 400 mg daily. Complete hematologic remission was achieved in all patients within 1 month, and all patients became PCR-negative for *FIP1L1-PDGFRA* after a median of 3 months of treatment. Patients continuing imatinib remained PCR-negative during a median follow-up period of

Table 1
Rearranged tyrosine kinase genes involved in eosinophilic neoplasms

Tyrosine Kinase Gene	Prototypic Genetic Rearrangement	Chromosome Location of Tyrosine Kinase Gene	Rearrangement Detected by Standard Cytogenetics?	Diagnostic Assays	Comments
PDGFRA	FIP1L1-PDGFRA	4q12	No	F[a],P	Alternative PDGFRA fusion genes can be detected by standard cytogenetics (eg, gene partners BCR, ETV6, KIF5B, CDK5RAP2, STRN, TNKS2, and FOXP1)
PDGFRB	ETV6-PDGFRB	5q31~33	Yes	C,F,P	More than 30 fusion PDGFRB partners have been described
FGFR1	ZMYM2-FGFR1	8p11~12	Yes	C,F,P	14 fusion partners of FGFR1 have been described
JAK2	PCM1-JAK2	9p24	Yes	C,F,P	Additional variants include ETV6-JAK2 and BCR-JAK2
FLT3	ETV6-FLT3	13q12	Yes	C,F,P	Other variants include SPTBN1-FLT3, GOLGB1-FLT3, and TRIP11-FLT3[b]
ABL1	ETV6-ABL1	9q34	Yes[c]	C[c],F[c],P,R	The ETV6-ABL1 variant can present with acute and chronic myeloid/ lymphoid phenotypes; eosinophilia more commonly accompanies myeloid disease

Abbreviations: C, standard cytogenetics; F, fluorescence in situ hybridization (FISH); P, reverse-transcriptase polymerase chain reaction; R, RNA-seq.

[a] FISH for the CHIC2 deletion is used to diagnose the FIP1L1-PDGFRA fusion.

[b] Chung et al. Cancer Genetics, in press; 2017.

[c] ETV6-ABL1 can result from complex rearrangements, including cryptic insertions; routine karyotyping can be inconclusive and FISH can miss small insertions.

Table 2
Activity of currently used tyrosine kinase inhibitors for myeloid/lymphoid neoplasms with eosinophilia

Rearranged Tyrosine Kinase Gene	Tyrosine Kinase Inhibitors in Use	Efficacy	Risk for Resistance/Progression/Death
PDGFRA	Imatinib	+++	Very low
PDGFRB	Imatinib	+++	Very low
FGFR1	Ponatinib Midostaurin	+	High
JAK2	Ruxolitinib	++	Variable
FLT3	Sorafenib Sunitinib Midostaurin	+/++	High
ABL1	Imatinib Nilotinib Dasatinib	++	Variable

+, low; ++, moderate; +++, high.
Modified from Reiter A, Gotlib J. Myeloid neoplasms with eosinophilia Blood 2017;129(6):711; with permission.

19 months. Another study prospectively assessed the natural history of molecular responses to imatinib doses of 100 to 400 mg daily.[11] Among 11 patients with high pretreatment transcript levels, all achieved a 3-log reduction in transcript levels by 1 year of therapy, and 9 of 11 patients achieved a molecular remission. In a long-term follow-up analysis of the Mayo cohort of 18 imatinib-treated *FIP1L1-PDGFRA*–positive patients, 1 patient with accelerated disease at presentation transformed to AML, but the median survival of the entire cohort was not reached and the otherwise excellent clinical outcomes confirmed the results of other studies.[15]

Discontinuation of imatinib in *FIP1L1-PDGFRA*–positive disease can lead to relapse. In a dose de-escalation trial of imatinib in 5 patients who had achieved a stable hematologic and molecular remission at 300 to 400 mg daily for at least 1 year, molecular relapse was observed in all patients after 2 to 5 months of either dose imatinib reduction or discontinuation.[18] Molecular remissions could be reestablished with reinduction of imatinib in all cases at a dose range of 100 to 400 mg daily. Hematologic relapse was noted only several weeks after discontinuation of imatinib in 4 patients in a Mayo study.[19] In the French series, imatinib was stopped in 11 patients; 6 of the patients subsequently relapsed, but 5 remained in persistent complete hematologic or molecular remission (range, 9–88 months).[16] In 2 patients with undetectable *FIP1L1-PDGFRA* transcripts by PCR for 4 years, no evidence of disease was detected for more than 2 years after discontinuation of imatinib.[20] In aggregate, these data suggest that imatinib can effectively suppress, but not eliminate the *FIP1L1-PDGFRA* clone in most patients; however, some individuals, particularly those with a longstanding complete molecular remission, may be able to achieve a cure after imatinib discontinuation. Similar to current guidelines in CML, ongoing imatinib treatment is recommended for *FIP1L1-PDGFRA*–positive disease.

Acquired resistance to imatinib is uncommon, with now more than 13 years of experience treating *FIP1L1-PDGFRA*–positive neoplasms.[7,21–26] Most cases occur in the blast phase of the disease and are usually due to a T674I mutation within the ATP-binding domain of PDGFRα. The T674I mutation is analogous to the T315I *BCR-ABL1* mutation in CML that confers resistance to imatinib, dasatinib, and nilotinib.[27]

Sorafenib elicited a transient response in a patient with the *FIP1L1-PDGFRA* T674I mutation in blast crisis, but was rapidly followed by a pan-resistant *FIP1L1-PDGFRA* D842V mutation.[23] Although sorafenib, midostaurin, and nilotinib demonstrate nano-molar inhibitory activity against the T674I mutant in vitro, these drugs have surprisingly limited clinical efficacy.[24–26,28] Ponatinib, which is the only currently approved TKI with activity against *BCR-ABL1* T315I, has also demonstrated potent in vitro activity against the *FIP1L1-PDGFRA* T674I and D842V mutants.[29,30] DCC-2036, a switch control inhibitor with activity against *BCR-ABL1* T315I, also has activity against cells expressing FIP1L1-PDGFRα T674I.[31] One report of primary resistance to imatinib was identified in a patient carrying tandem *FIP1L1-PDGFRA* S601P and L629P mutations.[32] Similar to recent in vitro findings with a *FIP1L1-PDGFRA* F604S mutation, the L629P mutation may induce resistance to imatinib by increasing stability of the fusion oncoprotein rather than interfering with drug binding.[33]

In patients with rearrangements of *PDGFRB* or *PDGFRA* fusions other than *FIP1L1-PDGFRA*, imatinib doses of 100 to 400 mg daily can elicit durable hematologic and cytogenetic remissions.[34–36] Long-term follow-up (median 10.2 years) of *PDGFRB*-rearranged patients treated with imatinib for a median duration of 6.6 years showed a 96% response rate and a 10-year overall survival (OS) rate of 90%.[36] None of the patients who achieved a complete cytogenetic or molecular remission lost their response or exhibited progression to blast crisis. In patients who present with *PDGFRA*-positive or *PDGFRB*-positive blast-phase disease or sarcoma, imatinib monotherapy produces durable complete and hematologic remissions (**Fig. 1**), whereas the experience with intensive chemotherapy and/or allogeneic stem cell transplantation (SCT), albeit very limited, has been disappointing.[37] The combination of TKI with intensive chemotherapy, similar to that undertaken with *BCR-ABL1*–positive acute lymphoblastic leukemia (ALL), requires exploration in future trials.

FGFR1 Fusion Genes

Patients with fusions involving the *FGFR1* gene exhibit karyotypes with a breakpoint involving chromosome 8p11. Fourteen *FGFR1* partners have been described to date; the most common reciprocal translocations include t(8;13) (p11;q12), t(8;9) (p11;q33), and t(6;8) (q27;p11), resulting in fusions of *ZMYM2, CNTRL,* and *FGFR1OP*, respectively, to *FGFR1* (see **Table 1**).[38–40] These diseases can present as a chronic myeloid neoplasm (usually an MPN) with variable eosinophilia, as de novo AML without an antecedent MPN, or as a B-cell or (more commonly) T-cell leukemia/lymphoma.[1,41] The disease follows an aggressive course usually terminating in AML (and/or less commonly B-cell ALL) in 1 to 2 years.[41] Therefore, intensive chemotherapy with regimens such as hyper-CVAD (cyclophosphamide, vincristine, doxorubicin [Adriamycin], and dexamethasone) (directed to treatment of T-cell or B-cell lymphoma), followed by early allogeneic transplantation, is recommended for patients who present with, or progress to, blast-phase disease.[41,42]

The data for use of small molecule inhibitors for patients with *FGFR1*-rearranged disease is sparse, but continually evolving (see **Table 2**). Midostaurin inhibited the *ZNF198-FGFR1* fusion in vitro, and elicited a hematologic (but not cytogenetic) response in a patient with this fusion.[43] Although *FGFR1* fusions are generally resistant to imatinib, nilotinib, and dasatinib, preclinical data indicate that ponatinib can inhibit the proliferation of, and induce apoptosis of, *FGFR1*-transformed cells.[44] Ponatinib was used as monotherapy and subsequently combined with induction chemotherapy (eg, hyper-CVAD) as a bridge to allogeneic hematopoietic SCT (HSCT) in a patient with a *BCR-FGFR1*–positive trilineage mixed phenotype acute leukemia.[45] Because of molecular persistence of *BCR-FGFR1* transcripts after transplantation, ponatinib was

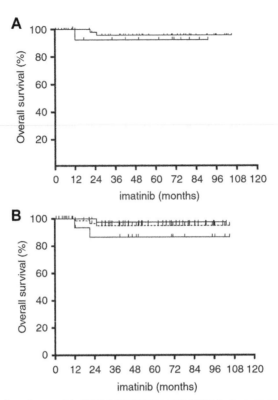

Fig. 1. Survival of patients with *FIP1L1-PDGFRA* or *PDGFRB* fusion genes with chronic or blast-phase disease. In (*A*), the upper curve represents the OS of 49 patients with *FIP1L1-PDGFRA* with chronic or blast-phase disease, and the lower survival curve represents the OS of 14 patients with diverse *PDGFRB* fusions. There is no statistically significant difference between the 2 survival curves. (*B*) The OS of all 63 patients (*middle curve*) with an *FIP1L1-PDGFRA* gene (n = 49) or diverse *PDGFRB* fusion genes (n = 14). Patients with chronic phase disease (*FIP1L1-PDGFRA*, n = 36; *PDGFRB* fusion genes, n = 10) are shown in the upper curve, and patients with blast-phase disease are shown in the lower curve (*FIP1L1-PDGFRA*, n = 13; *PDGFRB* fusion genes, n = 4). There are no statistically significant differences in survival among the 3 groups. (*From* Metzgeroth G, Schwaab J, Gosenca D, et al. Long-term follow-up of treatment with imatinib in eosinophilia-associated myeloid/lymphoid neoplasms with PDGFR rearrangements in blast phase. Leukemia 2013;27:2255; with permission.)

reintroduced at a dosage of 15 to 30 mg daily, resulting in disease-free survival now more than 3 years [45](Jason Gotlib, unpublished follow-up, 2017). Kreil and colleagues[46] evaluated the efficacy of ponatinib in 7 *FGFR1*-rearranged patients. In their series, ponatinib-treated patients demonstrated either progressive disease or unsustained hematologic or cytogenetic responses, similar to the results with intensive chemotherapy. Four patients who underwent allogeneic HSCT and achieved a CMR were alive after a median time of 19 months (range, 8–36) after diagnosis and 13 months (range, 4–29) after transplantation. Although allogeneic HSCT is currently the most promising option to achieve long-term remission or cure in patients with *FGFR1* fusions, the incorporation of FGFR1 inhibitors in the peritransplant setting may be a useful strategy for selected individuals that requires future validation.

Targeting the Janus Kinase/Signal Transducers and Activators of Transcription Pathway in Eosinophilic Neoplasms

The JAK1/JAK2 inhibitor ruxolitinib is approved for patients with intermediate and high-risk myelofibrosis, and in hydroxyurea-resistant or intolerant patients with polycythemia vera. Ruxolitinib and other JAK inhibitors are not specific to mutated JAK2; their activity relates to blockade of the JAK–signal transducers and activators of transcription (STAT) pathway, which can be activated not only by JAK2 V617F, but also by *MPL* and *CALR* driver mutations.[47] The clinical benefit from JAK-STAT inhibition in myelofibrosis manifests as reduction in disease-related symptoms and splenomegaly.[48,49] Rapid reduction in proinflammatory cytokines,[50] related to inhibition of inflammatory signaling cascades downstream of JAK1, is one mechanism underlying the clinical benefit of JAK inhibitors.

Infrequently, patients with idiopathic hypereosinophilic syndrome/chronic eosinophilic leukemia harbor *JAK2* V617F.[51,52] The JAK2-STAT pathway mediates antiapoptosis signals in eosinophils in response to granulocyte-macrophage colony-stimulating factor and interleukin-5,[53] as well as FIP1L1-PDGFRα.[54] Dysregulation of JAK2 kinase activity also results from fusions involving the *JAK2* gene. In the revised 2016 WHO classification, *PCM1-JAK2* has been added as a provisional variant to myeloid/lymphoid neoplasms with eosinophilia and abnormalities of *PDGFRA*, *PDGFRB*, and *FGFR1*.[1] Cases with *PCM1-JAK2* typically present as a chronic myeloid neoplasm with eosinophilia and marrow fibrosis; these are aggressive neoplasms with a natural history characterized by rapid progression to AML, and sometimes lymphoid blast crisis.[55–57] *BCR-JAK2* and *ETV6-JAK2* are rare variants of *PCM1-JAK2*, and may sometimes present with a phenotype similar to *BCR-ABL1*-like ALL.[58–61]

Ruxolitinib has been reported in a few cases of JAK2-rearranged disease. In 1 patient with chronic eosinophilic leukemia (CEL), ruxolitinib achieved a complete cytogenetic response[62]; in an initial and follow-up report of 2 patients with CEL, ruxolitinib produced complete hematologic and cytogenetic remissions, as well as marked reduction of *PCM1-JAK2* transcripts at 33 and 46 months after start of therapy at the time of reporting.[63,64] Schwaab and colleagues[65] treated 2 patients with a chronic myeloid neoplasm (one with *PCM1-JAK2* fusion and another with *BCR-JAK2* fusion gene) with ruxolitinib. After 12 months of therapy, both patients achieved a complete clinical, hematologic, and cytogenetic response. However, remission was short-lived in both cases; relapse occurred after 18 and 24 months, respectively, necessitating allogeneic HSCT in both patients.

FMS-like Tyrosine Kinase 3 Fusion Genes

Although internal tandem duplications (and less frequently, tyrosine kinase point mutations) in *FLT3* are common in AML, *FLT3* gene fusions are exceedingly rare in hematolymphoid neoplasms. Among the handful of cases described, *ETV6-FLT3* is by far the most common rearrangement.[66,67] *FLT3*-rearranged cases exhibit features of an eosinophilia-associated myeloid and/or lymphoid neoplasm, the latter usually manifesting as a peripheral T-cell lymphoma or T-lymphoblastic lymphoma. Multikinase small molecule inhibitors with activity against FLT3 have demonstrated modest activity and limited durability in patients with *FLT3* rearrangements. In 2 cases of *ETV6-FLT3*–positive CEL, sunitinib elicited complete hematologic and/or cytogenetic responses; however, responses were short-term and quickly followed by disease progression.[68] Falchi and colleagues[69] described a patient with *ETV6-FLT3*–positive CEL who achieved a complete hematologic and partial cytogenetic remission with sorafenib within 2 months of treatment. The patient was bridged to a matched sibling HSCT, and was in remission 11 months after initial diagnosis. The optimal role of such drugs, including newer agents with greater selectivity and potency against FLT3, may lie in their ability to maintain disease control in patients who are awaiting potential curative therapy with HSCT.[70]

SYSTEMIC MASTOCYTOSIS

SM encompasses a spectrum of subtypes from indolent SM (ISM), where OS is similar to age-matched controls, to advanced SM, which is an umbrella term for 3 variants: aggressive SM (ASM), SM with an associated hematologic neoplasm (SM-AHN), and mast cell leukemia (MCL).[71] The median OS for these 3 variants is 3.5 years, 2 years, and less than 6 months, respectively.[72,73] ASM is defined by 1 or more signs of organ damage due to neoplastic mast cell infiltrates.[71] In SM-AHN, the associated disease is almost always a myeloid neoplasm, such as myelodysplastic syndrome (MDS), myeloproliferative neoplasm, or an MDS/MPN overlap disorder, such as chronic myelomonocytic leukemia, CEL, or AML.[74]

In ISM, therapy is geared to control of mediator symptoms (eg, flushing, diarrhea, and anaphylaxis) with agents such as antihistamines, leukotriene antagonists, cromolyn sodium, and epinephrine on demand. In patients with advanced SM, small, retrospective studies of the cytoreductive agents pegylated (PEG)-interferon-α or cladribine (2-chloro-deoxyadenosine) have shown modest ability to reduce or reverse SM-related organ damage (reviewed in Ref.[75]). Although determination of the mutation status in the *KIT* gene (**Fig. 2**) is an essential component of the diagnosis of SM, it also guides selection of therapy because the mutational profile of *KIT* has implications for selection of specific TKIs (**Fig. 3**). Moreover, because the *KIT* D816 V mutation can be found in cells from both the SM and AHN,[76] selective inhibitors may prove efficacious in both disease compartments. The trial experience with inhibitors with activity against wild-type or D816V-mutated *KIT* is discussed in the following section.

Dasatinib and Nilotinib

Although dasatinib exhibits in vitro activity against KIT D816V,[77,78] a case series and a phase II trial of the drug (140 mg total daily dose) have shown limited activity in SM.[79,80] In a phase II trial of 33 patients with ISM and advanced SM, 11 (33%) responded.[80] Two complete responses were recorded in patients without the *KIT* D816V mutation, including a patient with *JAK2* V617F-positive SM with associated primary myelofibrosis (SM-PMF), and a patient with SM and concurrent CEL (SM-CEL). The other 9 responses were of a symptomatic nature only, without clinically significant reductions in either bone marrow mast cell burden or serum tryptase levels. Nilotinib was evaluated in an open-label phase 2 trial of 61 patients with SM; among the 37 patients with ASM, the overall response rate was 22%, and were no complete responses.[81]

Imatinib

Imatinib is approved by the Food and Drug Administration (FDA) for adult patients with aggressive systemic mastocytosis without the KIT D816V mutation or with *KIT* mutation status unknown. Imatinib lacks activity against KIT D816V in vitro and in vivo,[82,83] but it has demonstrated clinical benefit in patients with alternative *KIT* mutations or wild-type *KIT*.[84,85] For example, imatinib has elicited excellent responses in cases of the well-differentiated SM variant with either the F522C transmembrane *KIT* mutation[86] or wild-type *KIT*[87]; in a patient with familial SM carrying the germline *KIT* K509I mutation[88]; with deletion of codon 419 in exon 8 of *KIT* in pediatric CM[89]; and in a case of MCL with mutation in exon 9 (p.A502_Y503dup) (see **Fig. 2**).[90] In the context of SM, imatinib-sensitive mutations generally reside in exons 8 to 10 of the *KIT* gene, which include the juxtamembrane and transmembrane domains.

Masitinib

Masitinib (AB1010), an inhibitor of Lyn, Fyn, PDGFR-α/β, and *wild-type* KIT,[91] is approved in veterinary medicine for the treatment of unresectable canine mast cell tumors.[92] Lyn and Fyn are mast cell signaling molecules implicated in mediator release in mast cells, independent of *KIT* mutational status. Masitinib has been evaluated in phase II trials of patients with ISM or cutaneous mastocytosis with symptom handicap unresponsive to prior therapy.[93,94] The results of a phase III trial, randomized double-blind trial of masitinib versus placebo in patients with ISM and smoldering SM (80% of patients met formal criteria for SM) with symptom handicap were recently published.[95] Patients received oral masitinib (6 mg/kg daily) or placebo. The primary endpoint (eg, $\geq$75% improvement from baseline in at least 1 of 4 severe symptoms [pruritus, flushing, depression, or asthenia/fatigue]) was achieved by 19% and 7% of masitinib and placebo recipients, respectively. At week 24, there was a 20% absolute mean change in the serum tryptase level from baseline between the 2 groups in an intention-to-treat analysis: a decrease of 18% in the masitinib arm versus an increase of 2% in the placebo arm. In addition, urticaria pigmentosa lesions on masitinib therapy decreased by an average body surface area of 12% in the masitinib group and increased 16% in the placebo group. Masitinib-associated clinical benefits were generally sustained during a 2-year extension period. Excess adverse events observed with masitinib versus placebo included diarrhea, rash, and asthenia; in addition, masitinib was permanently discontinued in 24% of patients. The utility of masitinib in mitigating mediator symptoms will need to be weighed against the drug's adverse event profile in this patient population with otherwise low-risk disease.

Midostaurin

Midostaurin (N-benzoylstaurosporine; PKC412) is a multikinase inhibitor that demonstrates inhibitory activity against wild-type and D816V-mutated KIT, FLT3, PDGFR-α/β, and VEGFR2. In Ba/F3 cells transformed by *KIT* D816V, the IC_{50} (concentration of an inhibitor in which the response [or binding] is reduced by half) of midostaurin was 30 to 40 nM, compared with more than 1 μM with imatinib.[82,83] A partial response with midostaurin in a patient with MCL and an associated MDS/MPN,[83] and encouraging response rate of 69% in a phase 2 trial of 26 patients with advanced SM[96] led to a global, multicenter, open-label trial of midostaurin (100 mg twice daily on 28-day continuous cycles) in patients with ASM, MCL, and SM-AHN.[3]

The global trial used a steering committee and central pathology review to adjudicate eligibility, response, and histopathology. Among 89 evaluable patients, the overall response rate (defined as partial or complete resolution of 1 or more signs of organ damage related to SM) was 60%, of which 75% were major responses (MRs; defined by complete reversion of organ damage).[3] Responses were observed regardless of *KIT* D816V status, prior therapy, or the presence of an AHN. The median best reductions in serum tryptase level and bone marrow mast cell burden were −58% and −59%, respectively. Splenomegaly (evaluated by computed tomography or MRI volumetric imaging) decreased in 77% of evaluable patients. After a median follow-up of 26 months, the median duration of response (DOR) and median OS were 24.1 and 28.7 months, respectively. Median OS in responders was 44.4 months versus 15.4 months in nonresponders (hazard ratio for death, 0.42; $P = .005$). Of the 16 patients with MCL, 8 responded, including 7 MRs; among patients with MCL, the median

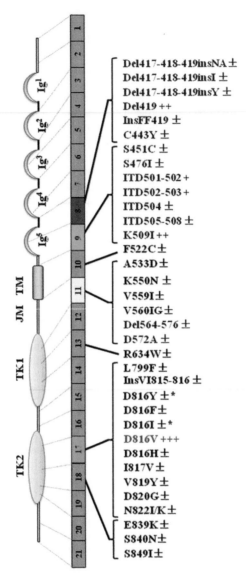

Fig. 2. Structure of the *KIT* gene and mutations in mastocytosis. Representation of the structure of KIT, illustrating the localization of the more frequently observed mutations in the *KIT* sequence in pediatric and adult patients with mastocytosis. The receptor is presented under its monomeric form, whereas its WT counterpart dimerizes upon ligation with stem cell factor (SCF) before being activated in normal cells. In children, the *KIT* D816V PTD mutant (in red) is found in nearly 30% of the patients, whereas the ECD mutants (in blue) are found in nearly 40% of the affected children, the most frequent being the deletion 419. In adults, depending of the category of mastocytosis, the *KIT* D81V mutant (in red) is found in at least 80% of all patients. The complete list of *KIT* mutants retrieved in the literature for mastocytosis is depicted here. In children, the structure of KIT is found WT in ~25% of the patients analyzed, whereas in adults, KIT is found WT in <20% of all patients analyzed so far. Some of the mutations are found only in a very few number of patients. Del, deletion; ECD, extracellular domain; Ins, insertion; ITD, internal tandem duplication; JM, juxtamembrane domain;

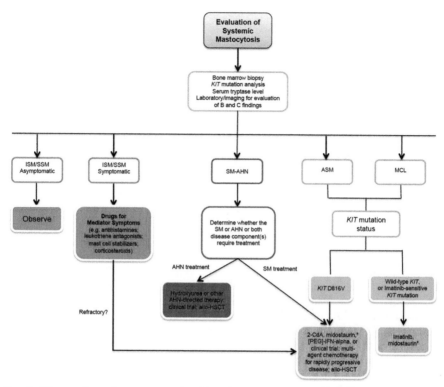

Fig. 3. Diagnostic and treatment algorithm for SM incorporating *KIT* mutation status. Workup of SM includes bone marrow biopsy, serum tryptase level, and *KIT* mutation status, to establish whether WHO diagnostic criteria for the disease are fulfilled. Evaluation is also focused on assessment of B and/or C findings (organ damage) and whether an AHN is present to establish the subtype of SM. Identification of the *KIT* D816 V mutation is not only a minor criterion for the diagnosis of SM, but is also important for stratifying potential treatment options. Imatinib is FDA-approved for adult patients with ASM without the *KIT* D816V mutation or with unknown *KIT* mutational status, and often exhibits efficacy against juxta-membrane/transmembrane *KIT* mutations. Midostaurin exhibits activity against KIT D816V and wild-type KIT. Additional selective KIT D816 inhibitors are currently in clinical trials. [a] Midostaurin is now FDA-approved for patients with ASM, SM-AHN, and MCL. (*Modified from* Ustun C, Arock M, Kluin-Nelemans HC, et al. Advanced systemic mastocytosis: from molecular and genetic progress to clinical practice. Haematologica 2016;101(10):1139; with permission.)

KI, kinase insert; PTD, phosphotransferase domain; TM, transmembrane domain; WT, wild-type. The symbols indicate the following: ±, mutation found in <10% of the pediatric or adult patients; +, mutations found in 1 to 5% of pediatric patients; ++, mutation found in 5 to 20% of pediatric patients; +++, mutation found in ~30% of pediatric patients and in >80% of all adult patients. *Mutation also found in children at low frequency. (*From* Arock M, Sotlar K, Akin C, et al. KIT mutation analysis in mast cell neoplasms: recommendations of the European Competence Network on Mastocytosis. Leukemia 2015;29(6):1225; with permission.)

DOR was not reached. The median OS was 9.4 months among all patients with MCL, and was not reached among responding patients with MCL. Symptoms and quality of life, measured by the Memorial Symptom Assessment Scale and Short-Form 12 survey, respectively, were significantly improved with midostaurin treatment. The ability of midostaurin to improve organ damage and symptoms may relate to its combined inhibitory effects on mast cell proliferation and immunoglobulin E–dependent mediator release.[97]

Midostaurin was generally well tolerated with a manageable toxicity profile consisting mostly of gastrointestinal side effects and myelosuppression, primarily in patients with preexisting cytopenias. These data support further exploration of midostaurin in combination with other agents with activity in advanced SM and in patients with ISM and refractory mediator symptoms. Midostaurin was approved by the FDA in April 2017 for the treatment of patients with ASM, SM-AHN, and MCL.

BLU-285

BLU-285 is a selective and potent inhibitor of KIT D816V signaling in preclinical models.[98] In the HMC1.2 cell line (both V560G and KIT D816V positive), BLU-285 blocks phosphorylation of AKT and STAT3, and in mice xenografted with P815 mastocytoma cells, the drug induced dose-dependent tumor inhibition.[98] Preliminary results of an ongoing phase 1 trial of BLU-285 in patients with SM have been reported recently.[99] Among 6 patients enrolled in the 2 lowest dosage cohorts of 30 to 60 mg daily, symptom improvement, weight gain, decrease of splenomegaly, and reductions of the serum tryptase and percentage of bone marrow mast cells have been observed. Thus far, the drug has been well tolerated in these initial dosing cohorts without reaching a maximum tolerated dose. BLU-285 and other KIT D816V-selective inhibitors in clinical development are attractive therapeutic options, given their restricted target profile, which may translate into less toxicity.

Targeting the Janus Kinase/Signal Transducers and Activators of Transcription Pathway in Systemic Mastocytosis

Although *JAK2* mutations are typically not found in SM except in rare cases in which a concomitant *JAK2* V617F-positive MPN is identified,[100,101] data indicate that wild-type JAK2 in important in mast cell activation and proliferation. JAK2 has been found to associate with KIT, and stem cell factor (SCF) binding to KIT induces increased JAK2 tyrosine kinase activity in human and murine cell lines and human progenitor cells.[102–104] Experiments with JAK2-deficient fetal liver cells revealed that SCF-induced growth and their differentiation into mast cells was markedly reduced, reinforcing the reliance on JAK2 for SCF signaling through KIT.[105] JAK2 is also a key regulator of FcεRI-mediated leukotriene production by mast cells.[106]

Experiments with the JAK2 inhibitor TG101348 revealed that it could reduce the proliferation of HMC1.2 cells bearing both *KIT* V560G and *KIT* D816V (IC_{50} 407 nm) with greater potency than HMC1.1 cells that carry only the *KIT* V560G mutation (IC_{50} 740 nM).[107] TG101348 inhibited the phosphorylation of JAK2 with IC_{50s} of 150 to 600 nM. Clinical experience with JAK inhibitors is limited to 2 case reports. In a patient with aggressive SM and a *KIT* 509I mutation who had persistent constitutional symptoms despite a complete morphologic response to imatinib, ruxolitinib abrogated persistent debilitating constitutional symptoms and improved cutaneous mast cell lesions.[108] Similar symptom improvement was observed with ruxolitinib in another patient with SM who also experienced reduction in splenomegaly and the leukocyte count, allowing the patient to transition to allogeneic HSCT.[109]

SUMMARY

Although imatinib generates outstanding responses in *PDGFRA* and *PDGFRB*-rearranged eosinophilic neoplasms, an unmet need exists for targeting other mutated TKs (eg, FGFR1, JAK2, FLT3), in which clinical benefit with currently available agents has proven to be less therapeutically tractable. The development of small molecule inhibitors with greater potency and selectivity against these targets is required. This strategy is being realized in advanced SM with midostaurin and novel KIT D816V inhibitors that are generating clinical impact in this historically challenging disease. Because the genetic complexity of these neoplasms often extends beyond singular lesions in TKs, combination therapy with drugs with different mechanisms of action or use of high-intensity procedures, such as allogeneic HSCT, should be evaluated on a case-by-case basis. In this regard, molecular annotation of patients with myeloid mutation panels will help inform the selection of tailored therapy.

REFERENCES

1. Arber DA, Orazi A, Hasserjian R, et al. The 2016 revision to the World Health Organization classification of myeloid neoplasms and acute leukemia. Blood 2016; 127:2391–405.
2. Arock M, Sotlar K, Broesby-Olsen S, et al. KIT mutation analysis in mast cell neoplasms: recommendations of the European Competence Network on Mastocytosis. Leukemia 2015;29:1223–32.
3. Gotlib J, Kluin-Nelemans HC, George TI. Efficacy and safety of midostaurin in advanced systemic mastocytosis. N Engl J Med 2016;374(26):2530–41.
4. Schaller JL, Burkland GA. Case report: rapid and complete control of idiopathic hypereosinophilia with imatinib mesylate. MedGenMed 2001;3:9.
5. Gleich GJ, Leiferman KM, Pardanani A, et al. Treatment of hypereosinophilic syndrome with imatinib mesilate. Lancet 2002;359:1577–8.
6. Ault P, Cortes J, Koller C, et al. Response of idiopathic hypereosinophilic syndrome to treatment with imatinib mesylate. Leuk Res 2002;26:881–4.
7. Cools J, DeAngelo DJ, Gotlib J, et al. A tyrosine kinase created by fusion of the PDGFRA and FIP1L1 genes as a therapeutic target of imatinib in idiopathic hypereosinophilic syndrome. N Engl J Med 2003;348:1201–14.
8. Griffin JH, Leung J, Bruner RJ, et al. Discovery of a fusion kinase in EOL-1 cells and idiopathic hypereosinophilic syndrome. Proc Natl Acad Sci U S A 2003;100: 7830–5.
9. Pardanani A, Ketterling RP, Brockman SR, et al. CHIC2 deletion, a surrogate for FIP1L1-PDGFRA fusion, occurs in systemic mastocytosis associated with eosinophilia and predicts response to imatinib mesylate therapy. Blood 2003;102: 3093–6.
10. Metzgeroth G, Walz C, Score J, et al. Recurrent finding of the FIP1L1-PDGFRA fusion gene in eosinophilia-associated acute myeloid leukemia and lymphoblastic T-cell lymphoma. Leukemia 2007;21:1183–8.
11. Jovanovic JV, Score J, Waghorn K, et al. Low-dose imatinib mesylate leads to rapid induction of major molecular responses and achievement of complete molecular remission in FIP1L1-PDGFRA-positive chronic eosinophilic leukemia. Blood 2007;109:4635–40.
12. Baccarani M, Cilloni D, Rondoni M, et al. The efficacy of imatinib mesylate in patients with FIP1L1-PDGFRalpha-positive hypereosinophilic syndrome. Results of a multicenter prospective study. Haematologica 2007;92:1173–9.

13. Klion AD, Robyn J, Akin C, et al. Molecular remission and reversal of myelofi-brosis in response to imatinib mesylate treatment in patients with the myelopro-liferative variant of hypereosinophilic syndrome. Blood 2004;103:473–8.

14. Helbig G, Moskwa A, Hus M, et al. Clinical characteristics of patients with chronic eosinophilic leukaemia (CEL) harbouring FIP1L1-PDGFRA fusion tran-script–results of Polish multicentre study. Hematol Oncol 2010;28(2):93–7.

15. Pardanani A, D'Souza A, Knudson RA, et al. Long-term follow-up of FIP1L1-PDGFRA-mutated patients with eosinophilia: survival and clinical outcome. Leu-kemia 2012;26:2439–41.

16. Legrand F, Renneville A, MacIntyre E, et al. The spectrum of FIP1L1-PDGFRA-associated chronic eosinophilic leukemia: new insights based on a survey of 44 cases. Medicine (Baltimore) 2013;92(5):e1–9.

17. Helbig G, Stella-Holowiecka B, Majewski M, et al. A single weekly dose of ima-tinib is sufficient to induce and maintain remission of chronic eosinophilic leukaemia in FIP1L1-PDGFRA-expressing patients. Br J Haematol 2008;141: 200–4.

18. Klion AD, Robyn J, Maric I, et al. Relapse following discontinuation of imatinib mesylate therapy for FIP1L1/PDGFRA-positive chronic eosinophilic leukemia: implications for optimal dosing. Blood 2007;110:3552–6.

19. Pardanani A, Ketterling RP, Li CY, et al. FIP1L1-PDGFRA in eosinophilic disor-ders: prevalence in routine clinical practice, long-term experience with imatinib therapy, and a critical review of the literature. Leuk Res 2006;30:965–70.

20. Helbig G, Kyrcz-Krzemień S. Cessation of imatinib mesylate may lead to sus-tained hematologic and molecular remission in FIP1L1-PDGFRA-mutated hyper-eosinophilic syndrome. Am J Hematol 2014;89:115.

21. Von Bubnoff N, Sandherr M, Schlimok G, et al. Myeloid blast crisis evolving dur-ing imatinib treatment of an FIP1L1-PDGFRalpha-positive chronic myeloprolifer-ative disease with prominent eosinophilia. Leukemia 2004;19:286–7.

22. Ohnishi H, Kandabashi K, Maeda Y, et al. Chronic eosinophilic leukaemia with FIP1L1-PDGFRA fusion and T674I mutation that evolved from Langerhans cell histiocytosis with eosinophilia after chemotherapy. Br J Haematol 2006; 134:547–9.

23. Lierman E, Michaux L, Beullens E, et al. FIP1L1-PDGFRalpha D842V, a novel panresistant mutant, emerging after treatment of FIP1L1-PDGFRalpha T674I eosinophilic leukemia with single agent sorafenib. Leukemia 2009;23:845–51.

24. Lierman E, Folens C, Stover EH, et al. Sorafenib is a potent inhibitor of FIP1L1-PDGFRalpha and the imatinib-resistant FIP1L1-PDGFRalpha T674I mutant. Blood 2006;108:1374–6.

25. von Bubnoff N, Gorantla SP, Thone S, et al. The FIP1L1-PDGFRA T674I mutation can be inhibited by the tyrosine kinase inhibitor AMN107 (nilotinib). Blood 2006; 107:4970–1.

26. Metzgeroth G, Erben P, Martin H, et al. Limited clinical activity of nilotinib and sorafenib in FIP1L1-PDGFRA positive chronic eosinophilic leukemia with imatinib-resistant T674I mutation. Leukemia 2012;26:162–4.

27. Bradeen HA, Eide CA, O'Hare T, et al. Comparison of imatinib mesylate, dasatinib (BMS-354825), and nilotinib (AMN107) in an N-ethyl-N-nitrosourea (ENU)-based mutagenesis screen: high efficacy of drug combinations. Blood 2006;108:2332–8.

28. Cools J, Stover EH, Boulton CL, et al. PKC412 overcomes resistance to imatinib in a murine model of FIP1L1-PDGFRalpha-induced myeloproliferative disease. Cancer Cell 2003;3:459–69.

29. Lierman E, Smits S, Cools J, et al. Ponatinib is active against imatinib-resistant mutants of FIP1L1-PDGFRA and KIT, and against FGFR1-derived fusion kinases. Leukemia 2012;26(7):1693–5.
30. Sadovnik I, Lierman E, Peter B, et al. Identification of ponatinib as a potent inhibitor of growth, migration, and activation of neoplastic eosinophils carrying FIP1L1-PDGFRA. Exp Hematol 2014;42(4):282–93.e4.
31. Shen Y, Shi X, Pan J. The conformational control inhibitor of tyrosine kinases DCC-2036 is effective for imatinib-resistant cells expressing T674I FIP1L1-PDGFRα. PLoS One 2013;29(8):e73059.
32. Simon D, Salemi S, Yousefi S, et al. Primary resistance to imatinib in Fip1-like 1-platelet-derived growth factor receptor alpha-positive eosinophilic leukemia. J Allergy Clin Immunol 2008;121:1054–6.
33. Gorantla SP, Zirlik K, Reiter A, et al. F604S exchange in FIP1L1-PDGFRA enhances FIP1L1-PDGFRA stability via SHP-2 and SRC: a novel mode of kinase inhibitor resistance. Leukemia 2015;29:1763–70.
34. Gotlib J. World Health Organization-defined eosinophilic disorders: 2015 update on diagnosis, risk stratification, and management. Am J Hematol 2015; 90(11):1077–89.
35. Cross DM, Cross NC, Burgstaller S, et al. Durable responses to imatinib in patients with PDGFRB fusion gene-positive and BCR-ABL-negative chronic myeloproliferative disorders. Blood 2007;109:61–4.
36. Cheah CY, Burbury K, Apperley JF, et al. Patients with myeloid malignancies bearing PDGFRB fusion genes achieve durable long-term remissions with imatinib. Blood 2014;123:3574–7.
37. Metzgeroth G, Schwaab J, Gosenca D, et al. Long-term follow-up of treatment with imatinib in eosinophilia-associated myeloid/lymphoid neoplasms with PDGFR rearrangements in blast phase. Leukemia 2013;27:2254–6.
38. Xiao S, Nalabolu SR, Aster JC, et al. FGFR1 is fused with a novel zinc-finger gene, ZNF198, in the t(8;13) leukaemia/lymphoma syndrome. Nat Genet 1998;18:84–7.
39. Guasch G, Mack GJ, Popovici C, et al. FGFR1 is fused to the centrosome-associated protein CEP110 in the 8p12 stem cell myeloproliferative disorder with t(8;9)(p12;q33). Blood 2000;95:1788–96, 2000.
40. Popovici C, Zhang B, Gregoire MJ, et al. The t(6;8)(q27;p11) translocation in a stem cell myeloproliferative disorder fuses a novel gene, FOP, to fibroblast growth factor receptor 1. Blood 1999;93:1381–9.
41. Bain BJ, Gilliland DG, Horny HP, et al. Myeloid and lymphoid neoplasms with eosinophilia and abnormalities of PDGFRA, PDGFRB, or FGFR1. In: Swerdlow S, Harris NL, Stein H, et al, editors. World Health Organization classification of tumours. Pathology and genetics of tumours of haematopoietic and lymphoid tissues. Lyon (France): IARC Press; 2008. p. 68–73.
42. Savage N, George TI, Gotlib J. Myeloid neoplasms associated with eosinophilia and rearrangement of PDGFRA, PDGFRB, and FGFR1: a review. Int J Lab Hematol 2013;35:491–500.
43. Chen J, DeAngelo DJ, Kutok JL, et al. PKC412 inhibits the zinc finger 198-fibroblast growth factor receptor 1 fusion tyrosine kinase and is active in treatment of stem cell myeloproliferative disorder. Proc Natl Acad Sci U S A 2004;101: 14479–84.
44. Chase A, Bryant C, Score J, et al. Ponatinib as targeted therapy for FGFR1 fusions associated with the 8p11 myeloproliferative syndrome. Haematologica 2013;98:103–6.

45. Khodadoust MS, Luo B, Medeiros BC, et al. Clinical activity of ponatinib in a patient with FGFR1-rearranged mixed phenotype acute leukemia. Leukemia 2016; 30:947–50.
46. Kreil S, Ades L, Bommer M, et al. Limited efficacy of ponatinib in myeloproliferative neoplasms associated with FGFR1 fusion genes (ASH Annual Meeting Abstracts). Blood 2015;126:2812.
47. Rampal R, Al-Shahrour F, Abdel-Wahab O, et al. Integrated genomic analysis illustrates the central role of JAK-STAT pathway activation in myeloproliferative neoplasm pathogenesis. Blood 2014;123(22):e123–33.
48. Verstovsek S, Mesa RA, Gotlib J, et al. A double-blind, placebo-controlled trial of ruxolitinib for myelofibrosis. N Engl J Med 2012;366(9):799–807.
49. Harrison C, Kiladjian JJ, Al-Ali HK, et al. JAK inhibition with ruxolitinib versus best available therapy for myelofibrosis. N Engl J Med 2012;366(9):787–98.
50. Verstovsek S, Kantarjian H, Mesa RA, et al. Safety and efficacy of INCB018424, a JAK1 and JAK2 inhibitor, in myelofibrosis. N Engl J Med 2008;363(12): 1117–27.
51. Schwaab J, Umbach R, Metzgeroth G, et al. KIT D816V and JAK2 V617F mutations are seen recurrently in hypereosinophilia of unknown significance. Am J Hematol 2015;90:774–7.
52. Pardanani A, Lasho T, Wassie E, et al. Predictors of survival in WHO-defined hypereosinophilic syndrome and idiopathic hypereosinophilia and the role of next-generation sequencing. Leukemia 2016;30:1924–6.
53. Simon HU, Yousefi S, Dibbert B, et al. Anti-apoptotic signals of granulocyte-macrophage colony-stimulating factor are transduced via Jak2 tyrosine kinase in eosinophils. Eur J Immunol 1997;27:3536–9.
54. Li B, Zhang G, Li C, et al. Identification of JAK2 as a mediator of FIP1L1-PDGFRA-induced eosinophil growth and function in CEL. PLoS One 2012;7: e34912.
55. Reiter A, Walz C, Watmore A, et al. The t(8;9)(p22;p24) is a recurrent abnormality in chronic and acute leukemia that fuses PCM1 to JAK2. Cancer Res 2005; 65:2662–7.
56. Murati A, Gelsi-Boyer V, Adélaïde J, et al. PCM1-JAK2 fusion in myeloproliferative disorders and acute erythroid leukemia with t(8;9) translocation. Leukemia 2005;19:1692–6.
57. Bousquet M, Quelen C, De Mas V, et al. The t(8;9)(p22;p24) translocation in atypical chronic myeloid leukaemia yields a new PCM1-JAK2 fusion gene. Oncogene 2005;24:7248–52.
58. Peeters P, Raynaud SD, Cools J, et al. Fusion of TEL, the ETS-variant gene 6 (ETV6), to the receptor-associated kinase JAK2 as a result of t(9;12) in a lymphoid and t(9;15;12) in a myeloid leukemia. Blood 1997;90:2535–40.
59. He R, Greipp PT, Rangan A, et al. BCR-JAK2 fusion in a myeloproliferative neoplasm with associated eosinophilia. Cancer Genet 2016;209:223–8.
60. Duployez N, Nibourel O, Ducourneau B, et al. Acquisition of genomic events leading to lymphoblastic transformation in a rare case of myeloproliferative neoplasm with BCR-JAK2 fusion transcript. Eur J Haematol 2016;97:399–402.
61. Bain BJ, Ahmad S. Should myeloid and lymphoid neoplasms with PCM1-JAK2 and other rearrangements of JAK2 be recognized as specific entities? Br J Haematol 2014;166:809–17.
62. Lierman E, Selleslag D, Smits S, et al. Ruxolitinib inhibits transforming JAK2 fusion proteins in vitro and induces complete cytogenetic remission in

t(8;9)(p22;p24)/PCM1-JAK2-positive chronic eosinophilic leukemia. Blood 2012; 120:1529–31.

63. Rumi E, Milosevic JD, Casetti I, et al. Efficacy of ruxolitinib in chronic eosinophilic leukemia associated with a PCM1-JAK2 fusion gene. J Clin Oncol 2013; 31:e269–71.

64. Rumi E, Milosevic JD, Selleslag D, et al. Efficacy of ruxolitinib in myeloid neoplasms with PCM1-JAK2 fusion gene. Ann Hematol 2015;94:1927–8.

65. Schwaab J, Knut M, Haferlach C, et al. Limited duration of complete remission on ruxolitinib in myeloid neoplasms with PCM1-JAK2 and BCR-JAK2 fusion genes. Ann Hematol 2015;94:233–8.

66. Vu HA, Xinh PT, Masuda M, et al. FLT3 is fused to ETV6 in a myeloproliferative disorder with hypereosinophilia and a t(12;13)(p13;q12) translocation. Leukemia 2006;20:1414–21.

67. Hosseini N, Craddock KJ, Salehi-rad S, et al. ETV6/FLT3 fusion in a mixed-phenotype acute leukemia arising in lymph nodes in a patient with myeloproliferative neoplasm with eosinophilia. J Hematopathol 2014;7:71–7.

68. Walz C, Erben P, Ritter M, et al. Response of ETV6-FLT3-positive myeloid/lymphoid neoplasm with eosinophilia to inhibitors of FMS-like tyrosine kinase 3. Blood 2011;116(8):2239–42.

69. Falchi L, Mehrotra M, Newberry KJ, et al. ETV6-FLT3 fusion gene-positive, eosinophilia-associated myeloproliferative neoplasm successfully treated with sorafenib and allogeneic stem cell transplant. Leukemia 2014;28:2090–2.

70. Chonabayashi K, Hishizawa M, Matsui M, et al. Successful allogeneic stem cell transplantation with long-term remission of ETV6/FLT3-positive myeloid/lymphoid neoplasm with eosinophilia. Ann Hematol 2014;93:535–7.

71. Horny HP, Metcalfe DD, Bennet JM, et al. Mastocytosis. In: Swerdlow SH, Campo E, Harris NL, et al, editors. WHO classification of tumors of hematopoietic and lymphoid tissues. 4th edition. Lyon (France): IARC; 2008. p. 54–63.

72. Lim KH, Tefferi A, Lasho TL, et al. Systemic mastocytosis in 342 consecutive adults: survival studies and prognostic factors. Blood 2009;113(23):5727–36.

73. Georgin-Lavialle S, Lhermitte L, Dubreuil P, et al. Mast cell leukemia. Blood 2013;121(8):1285–95.

74. Sperr WR, Horny HP, Valent P. Spectrum of associated clonal hematologic non-mast cell lineage disorders occurring in patients with systemic mastocytosis. Int Arch Allergy Immunol 2002;127(2):140–2.

75. Pardanani A. Systemic mastocytosis in adults: 2015 update on diagnosis, risk stratification, and management. Am J Hematol 2015;90(3):250–62.

76. Sotlar K, Colak S, Bache A, et al. Variable presence of KITD816V in clonal haematological non-mast cell lineage diseases associated with systemic mastocytosis (SM-AHNMD). J Pathol 2010;220:586–95.

77. Schittenhelm MM, Shiraga S, Schroeder A, et al. Dasatinib (BMS-354825), a dual SRC/ABL kinase inhibitor, inhibits the kinase activity of wild-type, juxtamembrane, and activation loop mutant KIT isoforms associated with human malignancies. Cancer Res 2006;66(1):473–81.

78. Shah NP, Lee FY, Luo R, et al. Dasatinib (BMS-354825) inhibits KITD816V, an imatinib-resistant activating mutation that triggers neoplastic growth in most patients with systemic mastocytosis. Blood 2006;108(1):286–91.

79. Purtill D, Cooney J, Sinniah R, et al. Dasatinib therapy for systemic mastocytosis: four cases. Eur J Haematol 2008;80:456–8.

80. Verstovsek S, Tefferi A, Cortes J, et al. Phase II study of dasatinib in Philadelphia chromosome-negative acute and chronic myeloid diseases, including systemic mastocytosis. Clin Cancer Res 2008;14:3906–15.

81. Hochhaus A, Baccarani M, Giles FJ, et al. Nilotinib in patients with systemic mastocytosis: analysis of the phase 2, open-label, single-arm nilotinib registration study. J Cancer Res Clin Oncol 2015;141:2047–60.

82. Akin C, Brockow K, D'Ambrosio C, et al. Effects of tyrosine kinase inhibitor STI571 on human mast cells bearing wild-type or mutated c-kit. Exp Hematol 2003;31:686–92.

83. Gotlib J, Berube C, Growney JD, et al. Activity of the tyrosine kinase inhibitor PKC412 in a patient with mast cell leukemia with the D816V KIT mutation. Blood 2005;106:2865–70.

84. Droogendijk HJ, Kluin-Nelemans HJ, van Doormaal JJ, et al. Imatinib mesylate in the treatment of systemic mastocytosis: a phase II trial. Cancer 2006;107: 345–51.

85. Vega-Ruiz A, Cortes JE, Sever M, et al. Phase II study of imatinib mesylate as therapy for patients with systemic mastocytosis. Leuk Res 2009;33:1481–4.

86. Akin C, Fumo G, Yavuz AS, et al. A novel form of mastocytosis associated with a transmembrane c-kit mutation and response to imatinib. Blood 2004;103: 3222–5.

87. Alvarez-Twose I, Gonazalez P, Morgado JM, et al. Complete response after imatinib mesylate therapy in a patient with well-differentiated systemic mastocytosis. J Clin Oncol 2012;30:e126–9.

88. Zhang LY, Smith ML, Schultheis B, et al. A novel K509I mutation of KIT identified in familial mastocytosis—in vitro and in vivo responsiveness to imatinib therapy. Leuk Res 2006;30:373–8.

89. Hoffmann KM, Moser A, Lohse P, et al. Successful treatment of progressive cutaneous mastocytosis with imatinib in a 2-year-old boy carrying a somatic KIT mutation. Blood 2008;112:1655–7.

90. Mital A, Piskorz A, Lewandowski K, et al. A case of mast cell leukemia with exon 9 KIT mutation and good response to imatinib. Eur J Haematol 2011;86:531–5.

91. Dubreuil P, Letard S, Ciufolini M, et al. Masitinib (AB1010), a potent and selective tyrosine kinase inhibitor targeting KIT. PLoS One 2009;4:e7258.

92. Marech I, Patruno R, Zizzo N, et al. Masitinib (AB1010), from canine tumor model to human clinical development: where are we? Crit Rev Oncol Hematol 2014;91(1):98–111.

93. Paul C, Sans B, Suarez F, et al. Masitinib for the treatment of systemic and cutaneous mastocytosis with handicap: a phase 2a study. Am J Hematol 2010;85: 921–5.

94. Moura DS, Sultan S, Georgin-Lavialle S, et al. Depression in patients with mastocytosis: prevalence, features an effects of masitinib therapy. PLoS One 2011; 6:e26375.

95. Lortholary O, Chandesris MO, Livideanu CB, et al. Masitinib for treatment of severely symptomatic indolent systemic mastocytosis: a randomised, placebo-controlled, phase 3 study. Lancet 2017;389:612–20.

96. Gotlib J, DeAngelo DJ, George TI, et al. KIT inhibitor midostaurin exhibits a high rate of clinically meaningful and durable responses in advanced systemic mastocytosis: report of a fully accrued phase II trial (ASH Annual Meeting Abstracts). Blood 2010;116:316.

97. Krauth MT, Mirkina I, Herrmann H, et al. Midostaurin (PKC412) inhibits immuno-globulin E-dependent activation and mediator release in human blood basophils and mast cells. Clin Exp Allergy 2009;39:1711–20.
98. Evans EK, Hodous BL, Gardino A, et al. First selective KIT D816V inhibitor for patients with systemic mastocytosis (ASH Annual Meeting Abstracts). Blood 2014;124:3217.
99. Drummond M, DeAngelo DJ, Deininger MW, et al. Preliminary safety and clinical activity in a phase 1 study of BLU-285, a potent, highly-selective inhibitor of KIT D816V in advanced systemic mastocytosis (SM) (ASH Annual Meeting Abstracts). Blood 2016;126:477.
100. Sotlar K, Bache A, Stellmacher F, et al. Systemic mastocytosis associated with chronic idiopathic myelofibrosis: a distinct subtype of systemic mastocytosis associated with a clonal hematological non-mast cell lineage disorder carrying the activating point mutations KITD816V and JAK2V617F. J Mol Diagn 2008; 10(1):58–66.
101. Schwaab J, Schnittger S, Sotlar K, et al. Comprehensive mutational profiling in advanced systemic mastocytosis. Blood 2013;122(14):2460–6.
102. Linnekin D, Weiler SR, Mou S, et al. JAK2 is constitutively associated with c-Kit and is phosphorylated in response to stem cell factor. Acta Haematol 1996; 95(3–4):224–8.
103. Weiler SR, Mou S, DeBerry CS, et al. JAK2 is associated with the c-kit proto-oncogene product and is phosphorylated in response to stem cell factor. Blood 1996;87(9):3688–93.
104. Brizzi MF, Zini MG, Aronica MG, et al. Convergence of signaling by interleukin-3, granulocyte-macrophage colony-stimulating factor, and mast cell growth factor on JAK2 tyrosine kinase. J Biol Chem 1994;269(50):31680–4.
105. Radosevic N, Winterstein D, Keller JR, et al. JAK2 contributes to the intrinsic capacity of primary hematopoietic cells to respond to stem cell factor. Exp Hematol 2004;32(2):149–56.
106. Sur R, Hall J, Cavender D, et al. Role of Janus kinase-2 in IgE receptor-mediated leukotriene C4 production by mast cells. Biochem Biophys Res Commun 2009; 390(3):786–90.
107. Lasho T, Tefferi A, Pardanani A. Inhibition of JAK-STAT signaling by TG101348: a novel mechanism for inhibition of KITD816V-dependent growth in mast cell leukemia cells. Leukemia 2010;24(7):1378–80.
108. Yacoub A, Prochaska L. Ruxolitinib improves symptoms and quality of life in a patient with systemic mastocytosis. Biomark Res 2016;4:2.
109. Dowse R, Ibrahim M, McLornan DP, et al. Beneficial effects of JAK inhibitor therapy in systemic mastocytosis. Br J Haematol 2017;176(2):324–7.

The Development of FLT3 Inhibitors in Acute Myeloid Leukemia

Jacqueline S. Garcia, MD*, Richard M. Stone, MD

KEYWORDS

- *FLT3*-ITD • *FLT3*-TKD • AML • FLT3 inhibitors • *FLT3* mutation

KEY POINTS

- Patients with FMS-like tyrosine kinase 3 gene (*FLT3*)–in-frame internal tandem duplication (ITD)–positive mutant acute myeloid leukemia (AML) generally have a poor prognosis.
- Midostaurin, a multitargeted kinase inhibitor, may soon be routinely added to chemotherapy in newly diagnosed mutant FLT3.
- Newer, more-specific FLT3 inhibitors, including some that target both *FLT3*-ITD and *FLT3*–tyrosine kinase domain (TKD), are being aggressively evaluated.

INTRODUCTION

AML is a heterogeneous malignant clonal disorder with an overall incidence of 4.1 per 100,000 individuals.[1] The prognosis, although variable, is generally poor. Although the molecular landscape is complex, cytogenetics and mutations are critical pathophysiologic and prognostic features of AML that can influence therapy.[2,3] Mutations in *FLT3* are identified in approximately one-third of patients with de novo AML (previously untreated and not arising from prior myelodysplastic syndrome).[4] The *FLT3*-ITD mutation is an independent predictor of a higher relapse rate and worse overall survival (OS) even when accounting for other clinical features.[4] The prognosis is particularly poor in those with a high ratio of mutant *FLT3*-ITD to normal gene, termed *allelic ratio*.[5] Small molecule inhibitors of FLT3, which vary in potency and specificity, have modest nondurable single-agent antileukemia activity. A recent study suggests, however, that adding midostaurin, a nonspecific FLT3 inhibitor, to standard frontline chemotherapy in *FLT3*-mutated AML patients confers a survival benefit. Thus, at least one drug targeting the *FLT3*-ITD mutation may soon be approved. Ongoing investigation of FLT3 tyrosine kinase inhibitors (TKIs) alone and in combination with other drugs in various AML disease settings will hopefully lead to further improvement in survival.

Department of Medical Oncology, Dana-Farber Cancer Institute, Harvard Medical School, 450 Brookline Avenue, Dana 2058, Boston, MA 02215-5450, USA
* Corresponding author. 450 Brookline Avenue, Dana 2054, Boston, MA 02215-5450.
E-mail address: jacqueline_garcia@dfci.harvard.edu

Hematol Oncol Clin N Am 31 (2017) 663–680
http://dx.doi.org/10.1016/j.hoc.2017.03.002
0889-8588/17/© 2017 Elsevier Inc. All rights reserved.
hemonc.theclinics.com

FLT3 PATHWAY ACTIVATION IN ACUTE MYELOID LEUKEMIA

Although most cell types express the FLT3 ligand (FL), the FLT3 tyrosine kinase receptor is expressed on a narrow range of cells, particularly on the surface of normal hematopoietic progenitors and frequently on their malignant counterparts. In normal physiology, after binding to its cognate ligand (FL), FLT3 dimerizes and undergoes a conformational change, which exposes the ATP-binding pocket in the activation loop to ATP. Ligand-activated FLT3 next undergoes autophosphorylation and transduces downstream signals, which promotes cell growth and prevents apoptosis through various intermediaries, including RAS/RAF/MEK/extracellular signal-regulated kinase (ERK), signal transducer and activator of transcription 5 (STAT5), and phosphoinositide (PI3)-kinase.[6]

Blasts from one-third of patients with AML harbor a mutation in *FLT3* (termed, *class I mutations*) and the clinical impact of the lesion varies by its location. FLT3-ITD mutations are characterized by insertions of repeated base pairs ranging 3 to > 400 base pairs in size within the juxtamembrane region of the receptor. FLT3 point mutations in the tyrosine kinase domain (FLT3-TKD) result in single amino acid substitutions within the activation loop, which are found in 5-10% of patients with AML. Although both of these mutations lead to constitutive FLT3 pathway activation, each has a biologically distinct mechanism.[7–9] The presence of the ITD leads to weak autoinhibitory activity of the juxtamembrane domain, resulting in a conformational change that leads to a constitutively active state even in the absence of FL.[10] The *FLT3*-TKD mutations, with half occurring at aspartate 835 (D835Y) in the activation loop, result in blocking ATP and substrate access to the kinase domain when the receptor is inactive, thereby interfering with the inhibitory effect of the loop and resulting in constitutive FLT3 kinase activation.[11] Less frequent *FLT3*-TKD mutations include Y842C, K663Q, and V592A and those occurring in the juxtamembrane domain.

IMPACT OF FLT3 MUTATIONS ON PROGNOSIS

The presence of an *FLT3*-ITD mutation carries negative prognostic impact. Younger adults (<60 years old) with normal karyotype AML who are *FLT3*-ITD mutation positive have shorter remission duration and OS (but not an inferior complete remission [CR] rate) compared with those with normal karyotype AML without *FLT3* mutation.[4] Not all mutant *FLT3*-ITD AML patients, however, have similarly inferior prognosis. One modifying factor is the mutant-to–wild type (WT) allelic ratio; a high allelic burden (greater than 0.5 or 0.7) correlates with worse outcome.[5,12,13] Some, but not all, studies have suggested that a greater ITD size may have a worse prognosis.[14,15] Standard chemotherapy results in a long-term disease-free survival (DFS) of only 20% to 30%; thus, allogeneic hematopoietic stem cell transplantation (allo-HCT) is typically recommended in first CR (CR1). Although allo-HCT may not be a panacea for all AML patients with an *FLT3*-ITD mutation, relapse rates and OS are superior after allo-HCT compared with those after chemotherapy alone, especially for patients with a high mutant-to-WT allelic ratio (relapse-free survival, $P = .02$; OS, $P = .03$).[13,16,17] The prognostic impact of *FLT3*-D835 mutations, however, is more controversial.[17] Patients with *FLT3*-TKD mutation have a superior outcome compared with those with an *FLT3*-ITD mutation: no difference in CR rate, but a 2-fold difference in the estimated 3-year DFS (60% vs 31%, respectively; $P = .01$), independent of *NPM1* mutation status.[17]

CHALLENGES TO TARGETING FLT3

The molecular context in which *FLT3* mutations occur may affect the success of FLT3 inhibitor treatment. *FLT3* mutations commonly co-occur with other AML somatic mutations[3,18] and behave more like a proliferative rather than a landscaping or founder somatic gene mutation in disease pathogenesis.[19,20] At the time of relapse where 1 clone tends to dominate, patients with AML who retain the *FLT3* mutation often display higher mutant allelic burden than at diagnosis.[21] In vitro studies suggest that blasts with higher mutant allelic burden were more responsive to selective FLT3 inhibition compared with cases of a low mutant allelic burden,[22] suggesting a rational strategy might be to consider a more-specific and potent FLT3 inhibitor in the relapsed setting and a less-selective FLT3 inhibitor in the more oligoclonal upfront setting.

CLINICAL EVALUATION OF FLT3 INHIBITORS

Given the poor prognosis of patients with *FLT3*-ITD AML, participation in a clinical trial should be considered when possible. Results from clinical trials with FLT3 TKIs in AML in the relapsed and upfront treatment setting are summarized in **Tables 1** and **2**, respectively. Less-specific FLT3 tyrosine kinase receptor inhibitors that have multiple targets include lestaurtinib (CEP-701), midostaurin (PKC412), sorafenib (BAY 43-9006), and sunitinib (SU11248). More-specific and potent FLT3 inhibitors include quizartinib (AC220), gilteritinib (ASP2215), and crenolanib (CP-868-596). A timeline of FLT3 inhibitor development for AML is shown in **Fig. 1**.

RELAPSED/REFRACTORY ACUTE MYELOID LEUKEMIA STUDIES WITH SINGLE-AGENT FLT3 INHIBITORS
First-Generation FLT3 Inhibitors

Lestaurtinib
Previously known as CEP-701, lestaurtinib is an orally available indolocarbazole derivative that was initially identified as an inhibitor of the neurotropin receptor TrkA but was found to have potent in vitro activity against FLT3. Treatment with lestaurtinib demonstrated safety, tolerability, and clinical activity in a phase I/II clinical trial of 14 patients with refractory, relapsed, or poor-risk AML with *FLT3*-activating mutations. Five patients evidenced clinical activity manifested by peripheral blood blast reduction and transfusion independence, but no actual CRs were noted.[23] Lestaurtinib is highly protein bound, specifically to α_1-acid glycoprotein, which may preclude adequate FLT3 inhibition as observed on ex vivo plasma inhibitory assays.

Midostaurin
Previously known as PKC412 (N-benzoyl staurosporine), midostaurin is an orally bioavailable indolocarbazole derivative that is a multitargeted TKI. Preclinical studies with midostaurin showed inhibition of activated FLT3 in the nanomolar range, selective induction of G1 arrest, and promotion of apoptosis.[24] A phase II study of single-agent midostaurin (75 mg by mouth 3 times a day continuously) was evaluated in 20 patients with relapsed or refractory AML or myelodysplastic syndrome with an activating mutation in *FLT3*.[25] Midostaurin was generally well tolerated with more than half of the patients experiencing grade 1 to 2 nausea and vomiting, although 2 patients had fatal pulmonary events of unclear etiology; 14 of 20 patients (70%) had 50% or greater peripheral blast count reduction. Pharmacodynamic studies confirmed inhibition of FLT3 autophosphorylation in most responders. A subsequent phase IIB study tested midostaurin at randomized doses of 50 mg or 100 mg twice daily in 95 patients with relapsed or refractory AML/myelodysplastic syndrome regardless of *FLT3* mutation status.[26] In addition to a high rate of hematologic improvement (HI) and blast reduction, 1 patient on 100 mg twice-daily dose of midostaurin experienced a partial remission (PR).

Table 1
Selected relapsed and refractory acute myeloid leukemia clinical studies with FLT3 inhibitors

Drug, Reference	Patients	FLT3 Status	Phase and Treatment Regimen	Treatment Response
Lestaurtinib[23]	18 yo+	+ any *FLT3* mutation	I/II: L 40–80 mg po bid, single agent	• 5 of 17 patients with lowered PB blasts (including 1 with BM blasts <5%)
Lestaurtinib[43]	18 yo+	+ *FLT3*-ITD or + *FLT3* TKD	II: randomized to chemotherapy alone vs L 80 mg po bid after MEC or HiDAC	• ORR (CR + CRp): 26% (n = 29 of 112; chemo + lestaurtinib) vs 21% (n = 23 of 112; chemo alone); P = .35
Sunitinib[27]	18 yo+	+/– *FLT3* mutation	I: Su 50–75 mg po daily, single agent	• *FLT3*-mutated: 4 of 4 achieved morphologic response or PR • *FLT3 WT*: 2 of 10 achieved PR
Sunitinib[44]	60 y+	+ *FLT3*-ITD or + *FLT3* TKD	I/II: Su 25 mg po daily plus 7 + 3, 3 cycles of intermediate-dose AraC and maintenance × 2 y	• 59% with CR/CRi (n = 13 of 22, including 8 of 14 with *FLT3*-ITD and 5 of 8 with *FLT3*-TKD)
Sorafenib[29]	18 yo+	+/– *FLT3* mutation	I: randomized to Sor continuous or intermittent dosing, 100–400 mg po BID, single agent	• 1 of 42 had CR (*FLT3*-ITD positive)
Sorafenib[48]	18–60 yo	+/– *FLT3* mutation	I/II: Sor 400 mg po (qod vs daily vs bid) plus AraC and Ida induction, Sor plus consolidation and Sor alone for maintenance × 1 y	• Phase I: CR in 4 of 10 (40%) (3 of 7 with *FLT3* mutant and 1 of 3 with *FLT3 WT*) • Phase II: CR in 38 of 51 (75%) (12 of 12 with *FLT3*-ITD, 2 of 2 with *FLT3*-TKD, and 24 of 36 with *FLT3 WT*) • Median 1-y OS 74%
Midostaurin[26]	18 yo+	+/– *FLT3* mutation	IIB: M 50 mg or 100 mg po bid, single agent	• PR: 1 of 95 • HI: 36 of 92 (46% with *FLT3*-mutant (n = 16 of 35) and 35% with *FLT3 WT* (n = 20 of 57))

Quizartinib[33]	18 yo+	+/− FLT3 mutation	I: q 12–450 mg/d daily	• Any type CR in 13% (n = 10 of 76); PR in 17% (n = 13 of 76), including responses in 53% with FLT3-ITD positive and 14% in FLT3-ITD negative • Median duration of response 13.3 wk • Median survival 14.0 wk
Quizartinib[35]	18 yo+	+ FLT3-ITD mutation	II: randomized to q 30 mg/d or q 60 mg/d po daily	• CRc: 47% • Median OS for q 30 mg/d: 20.7 wk • Median OS for q 60 mg/d: 25.4 wk
Gilteritinib[41]	18 yo+	+/− FLT3 mutation	I/II: G 20–450 mg po daily	• ORR (CR + CRp + CRi + PR) in 49% of FLT3-mutated vs 12% of FLT3 WT • ORR 52% in FLT3-mutated patients on G 80 mg or higher doses with median OS of 31 wk and duration of response of 20 wk
Crenolanib[40]	18 yo+	+ any activating FLT3 mutation	II: Cre 200 mg/m²/d 3 times a day continuously	• ORR 47% (12% with CRi, 32% HI, and 3% MLFS) • Median EFS 8 wk and OS 19 wk • FLT3 inhibitor naive vs prior TKI exposure with a median OS 55 wk vs 13 wk (P = .027) and EFS 13 wk vs 7 wk (P<.001)

Abbreviations: 7 + 3, daunorubicin + AraC; AraC, cytarabine; bid, twice daily; BM, bone marrow; Chemo, chemotherapy; CRc, CR + CRp + CRi; Cre, crenolanib; G, gilteritinib; Ida, idarubicin; L, lestaurtinib; M, midostaurin; MLFS, morphologic leukemia-free state; PB, peripheral blood; PO, by mouth; q, every; Q, quizartinib; qod, every other day; Sor, sorafenib; Su, sunitinib; yo, years old.

Table 2
Selected upfront acute myeloid leukemia clinical studies with FLT3 inhibitors

Drug, Reference	Patients	FLT3 Status	Phase and Treatment Regimen	Treatment Response
Sorafenib[49]	18 yo+	+/− FLT3 mutation	II: Sor 400 mg po bid plus AraC + Ida for induction, Sor plus cytarabine for consolidation, and Sor alone as maintenance × 1 y	• CR in 79% (n = 49 of 61) and CRp in 8% (n = 5 of 61), including CR/CRp 95% (n = 18 of 19) and 84% (n = 36 of 43) with and without FLT3-ITD, respectively • Median OS: 29 mo • Median DFS: 13.8 mo
Sorafenib[50]	60 yo+	+/− FLT3 mutation	II: randomized to Sor 400 mg PO BID vs placebo after DNR + AraC, after cytarabine for consolidation and as maintenance × 1 y	Placebo vs sorafenib: • ORR (CR + CRi) 64 of 95 vs 57 of 102 (P = .34), respectively • EFS 7 m vs 5 m (HR 1.26; 95% CI, 0.94–1.70) • OS 15 m vs 13 m (HR 1.03; 95% CI, 0.73–1.44) • Sorafenib arm had higher 60-d mortality (P = .035) attributable to infections (P = .015)
Sorafenib[51]	60 yo+	+ FLT3-ITD or + FLT3 TKD	II: sorafenib 400 mg po bid days 1–7 plus 7 + 3, followed by Sor plus intermediate dose AraC for consolidation and Sor alone as maintenance × 1 y	• CR or CRi in 69% (n = 37 of 54) • 1 y observed OS: 62% for FLT3-ITD and 71% for FLT3-TKD • Favorable outcome (1-y OS) compared with historical controls for FLT3-ITD (62% vs 30%; P<.0001)
Sorafenib[52]	18–60 yo	+/− FLT3 mutation	II: randomized to Sor 400 mg po bid vs placebo after 7 + 3 for induction, after cytarabine for consolidation and as maintenance × 1 y	Placebo (n = 133) vs sorafenib (n = 134): • CR: 59 vs 60% • 3-y EFS 22% (95% CI, 13–32) vs 40% (HR 0.64; 95% CI, 0.45–0.91; P = .013) • No OS difference

Midostaurin[55]	18–60 yo	+/– FLT3 mutation	Ib: M 50–100 mg, po bid, either concomitantly or sequentially with 7 + 3, M with HiDAC consolidation and M alone as maintenance	• 100-mg cohort: CR 45% (n = 13 of 29, including 8 of 23 with FLT3 WT and 5 of 6 with FLT3-mutant) • 50-mg cohort: CR 80% (n = 32 of 40, including 20 of 27 with FLT3 WT and 12 of 13 with FLT3-mutant) • FLT3-mutant cohort: 1-y OS of 0.85 (95% CI, 0.65–1.0); 2-y OS of 0.62 (95% CI, 0.35–0.88); 1-y DFS of 0.50 (95% CI, 0.22–0.78) • FLT3 WT cohort: 1-y OS of 0.78 (95% CI, 0.62–0.93); 2-y OS of 0.52 (95% CI, 0.33–0.71) in FLT3 WT; 1-y DFS of 0.60 (95% CI, 0.39–0.81)
Midostaurin[56]	18–60 yo	+ any activating FLT3 mutation	III: M 50 mg po bid vs placebo after 7 + 3 for induction, after HiDAC for consolidation, and as maintenance	M vs placebo: • CR: 59% vs 54%; P = .18 • 5-y OS: median 74.7 mo vs 26.0 mo, HR 0.77 (1-sided; P = .007) • 5-y EFS: median 8.0 mo vs 3.0 mo, HR 0.80 (1-sided; P = .004)
Midostaurin[57]	18–70 yo	+ FLT3-ITD mutation	II: M 50 mg po bid after 7 + 3 for induction, after HiDAC for consolidation, and as maintenance after chemo or allo-HCT	• Overall CR 75% after induction

Abbreviations: 7 + 3, daunorubicin + AraC; AraC, cytarabine; bid, twice daily; Chemo, chemotherapy; DNR, daunorubicin; Ida, idarubicin; L, lestaurtinib; M, midostaurin; mo, months; Sor, Sorafenib; yo, years old.

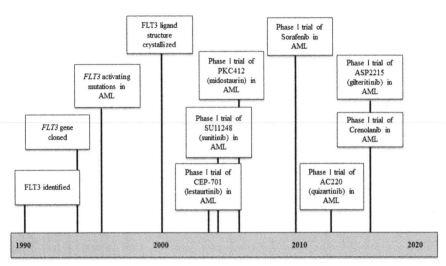

Fig. 1. History of FLT3 inhibitor therapy. A timeline of major scientific findings leading to the phase I clinical trials of first-generation and second-generation FLT3 inhibitors in AML.

Unlike other first-generation FLT3 inhibitors, midostaurin also has activity against FLT3 activation loop mutations.

Sunitinib

Previously known as SU11248, sunitinib (Sutent Pfizer, USA) is an oral, multitargeted receptor TKI approved in renal cell cancer whose multiple targets include vascular endothelial growth factor (VEGF), platelet-derived growth factor (PDGF), Kit, and FLT3. In a phase I clinical study of 15 patients with refractory AML, treatment with sunitinib alone led to short PRs in patients with *FLT3*-activating mutations (n = 4) and in 2 of 10 patients with WT *FLT3*.[27] Toxicities were significant, including 2 patients with fatal hemorrhage (although 1 had concomitant lung cancer) and several instances of grade 2 edema, fatigue, and oral ulcerations.

Sorafenib

The multikinase inhibitor sorafenib (BAY 43-9006 [Nexavar, Bayer, New Jersey]) is an orally bioavailable bis-aryl urea derivative approved for the treatment of metastatic renal cell cancer and advanced hepatocellular carcinoma. Although originally developed as an inhibitor of the serine/threonine kinase RAF, sorafenib also inhibits enzymes in various pathways, including RAS/RAF, c-KIT, VEGF receptor, PDGF receptor, and FLT3. This type II receptor TKI induces apoptosis in AML blasts and contributes to extracellular signal-regulated kinase (ERK) 1/2 inactivation and caspase-independent down-regulation of myeloid leukemia cell differentiation protein (Mcl-1).[28] Sorafenib alone in patients with relapsed/refractory AML was well tolerated at the continuous dose of 300 mg twice daily; 1 patient in a study with *FLT3*-ITD–mutated AML achieved a CR.[29] A simultaneous phase I study at the University of Texas M.D. Anderson Cancer Center explored sorafenib in a similar group of patients but determined the recommended phase II dose was 400 mg twice daily.[30] Dose-limiting toxicities (DLTs) included grade 3 or grade 4 hypertension, hyperbilirubinemia, and amylase elevation; 5 of 50 patients achieved CR or CR with incomplete platelet recovery (CRp). Responders were primarily had an *FLT3*-ITD mutation. Patients with *FLT3*-ITD mutations who did not respond had received prior FLT3 inhibitor treatment, suggesting a change in FLT3 addiction or the development of FLT3 inhibitor resistance. Potential expansion and emergence of the *FLT3*-D835 mutation during sorafenib therapy has been observed in mouse models transplanted with leukemia cells from patients before and after sorafenib therapy.[31] There was reduced expression of FLT3, phosphorylated FLT3, STAT5, and phosphorylated STAT5 in leukemic blasts before and after the development of sorafenib resistance, suggesting the presence of an alternative activation pathway.

Second-Generation FLT3 Inhibitors

Quizartinib

Formerly known as AC220, quizartinib is a more potent and selective inhibitor of FLT3 compared with the first-generation agents described previously. This type III receptor TKI has a 10-fold lower affinity for other receptor tyrosine kinases and is a more-selective FLT3 inhibitor with low nanomolar potency in cellular assays.[32] In a phase I study in 76 patients with relapsed/refractory AML, quizartinib demonstrated safety, tolerability, and preliminary efficacy.[33] Responses occurred in 23 of 76 patients (30%), including 10 (13%) CRs of any type. Furthermore, 9 of 17 *FLT3*-ITD–positive AML patients responded (53%; including 1 CR, 1 CRp, 2 CRs with incomplete count recovery [CRis], and 5 PRs) and 5 of 37 *FLT3*-ITD WT patients responded (14%; including 2 CRps and 3 PRs). Responses, however, were only durable for approximately 13.3 weeks. Common reported drug-related adverse events (mostly grade 2 or less) included nausea (16%), prolonged QT interval (12%), vomiting (11%), and dysgeusia (11%). The DLT was grade 3 QT prolongation. The maximum tolerated dose was declared 200 mg daily given continuously, although lower doses had promising efficacy without causing QT prolongation.[34] In vitro plasma inhibitor assays confirmed inhibition of *FLT3*-ITD phosphorylation at achievable concentrations. In the phase II setting, quizartinib alone led to an high overall response rate (ORR) with a composite CR rate of 47% and a median OS of 20.7 weeks for those on 30 mg/d and a median OS of 25.4 weeks for those on 60 mg/d.[35] Furthermore, in this and another phase II study, quizartinib successfully bridged one-third of patients with relapsed or refractory disease to transplantation; survival for these transplanted patients was only prolonged for an additional 2 months to 4 months compared with patients who were not transplanted on study.[36] Clinical durability may be limited by the development of resistance. The acquisition of secondary point mutations at residues within the kinase domain of FLT3 confers resistance or treatment failure with ITD-specific TKIs, including sorafenib[31] and quizartinib.[37] Although *FLT3*-ITD is a more common driver mutation, secondary TKD mutations represent critical additional targets.

Crenolanib

Unlike sorafenib and quizartinib, crenolanib besylate (formerly, CP-868,-596) is active against both the FLT3-D835 residue and FLT3-ITD, signifying its potency as a pan-FLT3 inhibitor with type I TKI properties.[38] Crenolanib also targets PDGF receptors α and β. Preclinical models of crenolanib have shown equal inhibition of WT and ITD-mutated FLT3 autophosphorylation with a half-maximal inhibitory concentration of approximately 2 nM in AML cells.[39] In a phase II study of crenolanib administered at 200 mg/m^2/day divided in three doses daily continuously in relapsed or refractory AML with activating *FLT3* mutations, the ORR at a median of 14 weeks' follow-up was 47% (including 12% CRi, 32% HI, and 3% morphologic leukemia-free state).[40] Patients who were TKI naive compared with those with prior TKI exposure were more likely to benefit from crenolanib therapy (median OS approximately 55 weeks vs 13 weeks, respectively; $P = .027$). Grade 3 toxicities included abdominal pain and nausea.

Gilteritinib

Also known as ASP2215, gilteritinib is a selective FLT3 and AXL inhibitor with activity against *FLT3*-ITD and *FLT3*-TKD. Final results from the Chrysalis Trial, a phase I/II clinical trial of gilteritinib in patients with relapsed or refractory AML that was enriched for *FLT3* mutations demonstrated significant single-agent clinical activity.[41] Most patients were heavily pretreated and had an *FLT3*-activating mutation (194 of 252 patients had an *FLT3* mutation, including *FLT3*-ITD, n = 159; *FLT3*-D835, n = 13; *FLT3*-ITD and *FLT3*-D835, n = 16; and other, n = 6). Common treatment-related adverse events included diarrhea (16%) and fatigue (15%); QTC prolongation (>500 milliseconds) was infrequently observed (<5%). Patients who had mutant *FLT3* disease had an ORR (including CR + CRp + CRi + PR) of 49% and those who were *FLT3* WT had an ORR of 12%. *FLT3*-mutated patients who were on a minimum of 80 mg daily (n = 169) had potent FLT3 inhibition by plasma inhibitory activity assays with an ORR of 52% and a median OS of 31 weeks (range 1.7–61 weeks).

Promising results from the early-phase clinical studies with these second-generation FLT3 inhibitors have led to the development of large, multicenter randomized phase III studies, including quizartinib versus salvage chemotherapy (QUANTUM-R study; NCT02039726) and gilteritinib versus salvage chemotherapy (NCT02421939). The QUANTUM-R study is a randomized clinical trial (2:1) with quizartinib versus salvage chemotherapy (investigator's choice: mitoxantrone, etoposide, and intermediate-dose cytarabine [MEC]; fludarabine, cytarabine, and granulocyte colony-stimulating factor with idarubicin [FLAG-IDA]; or low-dose cytarabine [LoDAC] for FLT3 TKI–naive patients with *FLT3*-ITD–positive AML in first relapse or refractory to prior therapy). The phase III, open-label, multicenter randomized study of gilteritinib versus salvage chemotherapy in adults with first relapse or primary refractory *FLT3* mutation–positive AML is another ongoing registration trial.[42] Patients must have an activating mutation in *FLT3* and are randomized 2:1 to treatment with either gilteritinib, 120 mg daily, or to investigator's prerandomization choice of prespecified salvage therapy. These trials will help to determine if more-selective FLT3 inhibitors offer a survival advantage compared with routine salvage chemotherapy, which could change current practice.

Summary of monotherapy with FLT3 inhibitors in acute myeloid leukemia

Second-generation FLT3 inhibitors have generated excellent response rates in relapsed/refractory AML patients with *FLT3* mutations. Overall, single-agent second-generation FLT3 inhibitors have demonstrated encouraging clinical activity that may or may not be high enough to justify approval. Combination with another agent(s), however, may increase their efficacy and magnify the impact on the outcome of patients with *FLT3*-activating mutations.

RELAPSED/REFRACTORY ACUTE MYELOID LEUKEMIA STUDIES WITH FLT3 INHIBITORS COMBINED WITH STANDARD THERAPIES

First-Generation FLT3 Inhibitors in Combination with Conventional Salvage Chemotherapy

Lestaurtinib

In the multicenter, randomized Cephalon 204 trial for patients with AML with an *FLT3* activating mutation in first relapse, salvage chemotherapy alone (either MEC or high-dose cytarabine [HiDAC] depending on duration of first remission) was compared with salvage chemotherapy followed by lestaurtinib administered 80 mg twice daily.[43] There was no difference in CR rate (21% vs 26%, respectively; P = .35) or in OS in either arm. Pharmacodynamic studies showed that *FLT3* inhibition at day 15 was only achieved in just over half of the patients on the lestaurtinib arm.

Sunitinib

In a phase I/II clinical trial for patients with relapsed or refractory AML regardless of *FLT3* mutation status, sunitinib was tested in combination with standard chemotherapy.[44] Results showed a combined CR and CRi rate of 59% (n = 13 of 22 patients). In particular, responders included 8 of 14 with *FLT3*-ITD mutation and 5 of 8 with *FLT3*-TKD mutation. DLTs included prolonged count recovery and hand-foot syndrome.

Second-Generation FLT3 Inhibitors in Combination with Conventional Salvage Chemotherapy

In addition to these studies, an open-label, dose de-escalation, phase Ib pilot study of crenolanib in combination with standard salvage chemotherapy for patients with relapsed or refractory AML irrespective of *FLT3* mutation status is under way (NCT02626338). Early results from a single-institution study idarubicin, at 12 mg/m^2/d for 3 days and HiDAC (cytarabine, 1.5 g/m^2/d over 3 hours for 4 days or 3 days if >60 years old) plus dose-escalated crenolanib starting on day 5 for relapsed/refractory *FLT3*-mutated AML showed that safety and tolerability when sorafenib was dosed at 100 mg 3 times a day.[45] The regimen allowed for the addition of crenolanib to postremission therapies, including consolidation and maintenance but not post–allo-HCT. The ORR in 11 evaluable patients to date was 36%, including 1 CR and 3 CRi. Remissions were not achieved in patients with prior FLT3 inhibitor exposure.

TREATMENT-NAIVE ACUTE MYELOID LEUKEMIA STUDIES WITH FLT3 INHIBITORS IN COMBINATION WITH CONVENTIONAL CHEMOTHERAPY
Lestaurtinib

This first-generation FLT3 inhibitor was investigated as a part of the UK AML 15 and AML 17 trials in patients with previously untreated AML with a confirmed *FLT3*-activating mutation[46]; 500 patients were randomized between lestaurtinib and control. The results were largely negative, demonstrating no overall clinical benefit with the addition of *FLT3*-directed therapy alongside upfront chemotherapy. This drug will not likely be further developed given its limited activity as a FLT3 inhibitor.

Sorafenib

Preclinical studies have shown synergistic activity when FLT3 TKIs were used simultaneously with or immediately after cytotoxic chemotherapy agents.[47] TKIs may be possibly antagonistic when administered prior to chemotherapy (TKI may prevent cell cycling and render S-phase–specific agents, such as cytarabine, ineffective). An initial phase I/II study showed safety and tolerability when combining sorafenib (400 mg twice daily for 7 days) to upfront chemotherapy in patients with previously untreated AML regardless of *FLT3* mutation status.[48,49] Of the 62 patients treated on study, 49 achieved CR (79%) and 5 achieved a CRp (8%), including 18 of 19 (95%) and 36 of 43 (84%) patients with and without *FLT3*-ITD, respectively. A study directed at patients 60 years and older led by the Study Alliance Leukemia group trial failed to demonstrate clinical benefit likely due to higher treatment-related mortality.[50] In contrast to prior studies, sorafenib was administered from day +3 after end of chemotherapy until 3 days prior to the next treatment course. Efficacy and tolerability were evidenced, however, with a 7-day sorafenib schedule in older patients with *FLT3*-mutated AML who participated in the Alliance C11001 phase II trial of sorafenib plus standard induction chemotherapy[51]; 36 of 54 evaluable patients (69%) achieved a CR or CRi with similar rates of response among those with *FLT3*-ITD and *FLT3*-TKD mutations. Screening for *FLT3* mutation status was feasible using a central laboratory (median turnaround time approximately 46 hours). A large, randomized, double-blind, placebo-controlled phase II study (SORAML) was next conducted to assess the benefit of adding sorafenib versus placebo to standard induction chemotherapy in newly diagnosed, previously untreated AML aged 60 years and younger regardless of *FLT3* mutation status.[52] At 36-month follow-up, the median event-free survival (EFS) was 9 months in the placebo cohort versus 21 months in the sorafenib cohort (hazard ratio [HR] 0.64; 95% CI, 0.45–0.91; P = .013). Those in the sorafenib cohort reported more frequent fever, diarrhea, bleeding, cardiac events, and hand-foot-skin reaction events. Induction mortality was similar to that previously reported with chemotherapy alone. Patients receiving sorafenib had a decreased risk of relapse and an increased duration of remission that was not restricted to patients with *FLT3*-ITD mutations; TKD mutations were not assessed. The benefits of adding sorafenib to standard chemotherapy were not restricted to *FLT3*-mutated AML, suggesting that it may clinically behave as a multitargeted kinase inhibitor rather than a specific FLT3 inhibitor. In summary, sorafenib in combination with chemotherapy seems well tolerated for younger patients with AML, but its role in patients 60 years and older remains unclear.

Quizartinib

Quizartinib was dosed sequentially after each of 2 courses of cytarabine, daunorubicin, and etoposide followed by 1 course of daunorubicin and cytarabine (2 + 5) in older patients with both mutant and WT *FLT3* untreated AML.[53] The addition of quizartinib was safe and tolerated. CR was achieved in 33 of 42 patients (79%; inciuing 4 patients with *FLT3*-ITD mutation). These positive findings will be further assessed in a phase III, randomized, double-blind, placebo-controlled global study of quizartinib with standard-of-care chemotherapy and as maintenance therapy in patients with untreated *FLT3*-ITD–positive AML (QUANTUM-First) (NCT02668653).[54]

Midostaurin

Positive findings from the phase Ib study[55] of midostaurin combined with intensive chemotherapy for patients with unselected AML led to the development of a randomized phase III clinical trial (RATIFY, Cancer and Leukemia Group B [CALGB] C10603)[56] for younger patients with *FLT3*-mutated AML, which was the first biomarker mutation–driven trial in AML with a positive OS benefit for patients randomized to midostaurin.[56] *FLT3* mutation status was obtained within 2 days to 3 days during screening. Treatment consisted of daunorubicin, 60 mg/m^2 intravenously (IV) days 1 to 3, and cytarabine, 200 mg/m^2 days 1 to 7 continuously by IV (3 + 7), plus midostaurin (50 mg by mouth twice daily) or placebo administered on days 8 to 22. Midostaurin or placebo was continued in addition to chemotherapy as postremission therapy for up to 4 cycles followed by 1 year of maintenance therapy. The positive OS benefit was appreciated in the overall analysis and when patients were censored at the time of CR for transplantation (HR = 0.77; P = .007). These results will likely change the current treatment paradigm for young patients with AML with an activating *FLT3* mutation. Positive data from an ongoing AMLSG single-arm, phase II, multicenter clinical trial (NCT01477606) for patients with untreated *FLT3*-ITD–mutated AML further demonstrated the feasibility and benefit of dose-adapted midostaurin when added to intensive induction chemotherapy and to maintenance therapy.[57]

Crenolanib

A phase II study of crenolanib in combination with standard induction chemotherapy in patients with AML with *FLT3*-activating mutations is ongoing (NCT02283177).[58]

Preliminary results from the first 26 evaluable patients (*ITD*-mutant, n = 19; D835-mutant, n = 3; and multiple *FLT3*-activating mutations, n = 4) who received 7 + 3 induction chemotherapy followed by crenolanib, 100 mg by mouth 3 times daily starting day 9, showed that the addition of crenolanib was tolerable and led to a high response rate (88% with CR after 1 cycle and 96% ORR [CR + Cri]). Crenolanib was also administered concurrently with consolidation therapy and as maintenance therapy for up to 1 year after HiDAC or allo-HCT. With a median follow-up of 6 months at time of analysis, the median OS was greater than 80%. Whether or not more-specific FLT3 inhibitors will have a bigger survival effect than midostaurin when combined with chemotherapy at diagnosis is still under investigation.

FIRST-GENERATION AND SECOND-GENERATION FLT3 INHIBITORS IN COMBINATION WITH HYPOMETHYLATING AGENTS

Hypomethylating agents are commonly offered to patients ineligible for intensive chemotherapy given overall tolerability and evidence of modest antileukemic activity.[59,60] Hypomethylating agents are hypothesized to induce lower levels of FL compared with intensive chemotherapy and thus less likely to generate resistance. In a phase I/II clinical trial for patients with relapsed or refractory AML with *FLT3*-ITD, azacitidine was administered at 75 mg/m^2 IV daily for 7 days and sorafenib at 400 mg twice daily continuously and repeated monthly.[61] A robust response rate of 46% (6 with CR [16%], 10 with CRi [27%], and 1 with PR [3%]) in 37 evaluable patients was observed. The median time to remission was approximately 2 cycles and the median duration of remission was 2.3 months. Plasma inhibitory assays showed adequate FLT3 inhibition (defined as >85%) in 64% of patients during the first cycle of therapy, which correlated with plasma sorafenib concentrations. Treatment was well tolerated with expected grade 3 or higher adverse events that were primarily hematologic, including neutropenia with fever or infection, and a 4-week treatment-related mortality rate of 9%. Azacitidine plus sorafenib may arguably be a sensible choice to consider in the salvage setting when clinical trials are not available for patients with *FLT3*-ITD–mutated AML.

Summary of FLT3 Inhibitors in Combination with Standard Chemotherapy

For patients with *FLT3* mutation–positive disease, the addition of midostaurin to standard chemotherapy evidenced an OS advantage compared with placebo in the RATIFY phase III clinical trial. The use of sorafenib may also be considered until midostaurin becomes commercially available given the EFS and relapse-free survival benefit noted in the SORAML trial. Furthermore, in the less-intensive treatment setting for patients with *FLT3*-ITD–mutated AML, azacytidine and sorafenib combination treatment is a suitable option. Whether any OS benefit can be enhanced by longer exposure or as maintenance after allo-HCT needs to be determined; early studies are described later.

ROLE FOR FLT3 INHIBITION AS MAINTENANCE THERAPY

Disease relapse is not uncommon in patients with *FLT3*-ITD–mutated AML even after allo-HCT. FL levels increase after chemotherapy-induced marrow aplasia, hence FLT3 inhibition during maintenance is a rational strategy.[62] Preclinical data have demonstrated that first generation inhibitors, such as sorafenib, can synergize with the alloimmune effects provided by the donor graft.[63] A phase I maintenance study of sorafenib treatment in patients with *FLT3*-ITD AML who were post–allo-HCT demonstrated that the addition of sorafenib (between days 45 and 120 post-transplant for up to 1 year) was safe and well tolerated. One patient experienced acute graft-versus-host disease (GVHD) and 38% of patients had evidence of any chronic GVHD during maintenance therapy.[64] The 1-year PFS rate was 85% (90% CI, 66%–94%) and 1-year OS was 95% (90% CI, 79%–99%) after transplant. Historically, patients with *FLT*-ITD AML have a high rate of relapse after transplant compared with patients who are *FLT3* WT (30% vs 16%, respectively).[16] These striking results suggest that sorafenib can potentially reduce the rate of relapse for patients with *FLT3*-ITD AML with acceptable GVHD risk. Quizartinib was also tested as maintenance in the post–allo-HCT setting for patients with *FLT3*-ITD AML with similar safety and tolerability.[65] A Blood and Marrow Transplant Clinical Trials Network trial will randomize *FLT3*-mutated AML patients to gilteritinib versus placebo to more formally evaluate the benefit of a specific FLT3 inhibitor in the post–allo-HCT maintenance setting.

SUMMARY

Personalized therapy is slowly becoming a reality for patients with AML, in particular for patients with *FLT3*-activating mutations. The treatment combinations that will ultimately provide optimal outcomes in terms of response duration and OS remain to be determined. Results from the RATIFY trial have provided a new standard of care for the treatment of younger patients with *FLT3*-mutated AML; the post-transplant studies have provided compelling evidence for using FLT3 inhibitors as maintenance therapy.

REFERENCES

1. NCI. SEER Stat fact sheets: acute myeloid leukemia (AML). Available at: https://seer.cancer.gov/statfacts/html/amyl.html. Accessed November 1, 2016.
2. Dohner H, Estey EH, Amadori S, et al. Diagnosis and management of acute myeloid leukemia in adults: recommendations from an international expert panel, on behalf of the European LeukemiaNet. Blood 2010;115(3):453–74.
3. Cancer Genome Atlas Research Network. Genomic and epigenomic landscapes of adult de novo acute myeloid leukemia. N Engl J Med 2013;368(22):2059–74.
4. Frohling S, Schlenk RF, Breitruck J, et al. Prognostic significance of activating FLT3 mutations in younger adults (16 to 60 years) with acute myeloid leukemia and normal cytogenetics: a study of the AML Study Group Ulm. Blood 2002; 100(13):4372–80.
5. Thiede C, Steudel C, Mohr B, et al. Analysis of FLT3-activating mutations in 979 patients with acute myelogenous leukemia: association with FAB subtypes and identification of subgroups with poor prognosis. Blood 2002;99(12):4326–35.
6. Rosnet O, Buhring HJ, deLapeyriere O, et al. Expression and signal transduction of the FLT3 tyrosine kinase receptor. Acta Haematol 1996;95(3–4):218–23.
7. Yamamoto Y, Kiyoi H, Nakano Y, et al. Activating mutation of D835 within the activation loop of FLT3 in human hematologic malignancies. Blood 2001;97(8): 2434–9.
8. Kiyoi H, Ohno R, Ueda R, et al. Mechanism of constitutive activation of FLT3 with internal tandem duplication in the juxtamembrane domain. Oncogene 2002; 21(16):2555–63.
9. Mead AJ, Linch DC, Hills RK, et al. FLT3 tyrosine kinase domain mutations are biologically distinct from and have a significantly more favorable prognosis than FLT3 internal tandem duplications in patients with acute myeloid leukemia. Blood 2007;110(4):1262–70.
10. Griffith J, Black J, Faerman C, et al. The structural basis for autoinhibition of FLT3 by the juxtamembrane domain. Mol Cell 2004;13(2):169–78.

11. Abu-Duhier FM, Goodeve AC, Wilson GA, et al. Identification of novel FLT-3 Asp835 mutations in adult acute myeloid leukaemia. Br J Haematol 2001; 113(4):983–8.

12. Whitman SP, Archer KJ, Feng L, et al. Absence of the wild-type allele predicts poor prognosis in adult de novo acute myeloid leukemia with normal cytogenetics and the internal tandem duplication of FLT3: a cancer and leukemia group B study. Cancer Res 2001;61(19):7233–9.

13. Schlenk RF, Kayser S, Bullinger L, et al. Differential impact of allelic ratio and insertion site in FLT3-ITD-positive AML with respect to allogeneic transplantation. Blood 2014;124(23):3441–9.

14. Stirewalt DL, Kopecky KJ, Meshinchi S, et al. Size of FLT3 internal tandem duplication has prognostic significance in patients with acute myeloid leukemia. Blood 2006;107(9):3724–6.

15. Ponziani V, Gianfaldoni G, Mannelli F, et al. The size of duplication does not add to the prognostic significance of FLT3 internal tandem duplication in acute myeloid leukemia patients. Leukemia 2006;20(11):2074–6.

16. Brunet S, Labopin M, Esteve J, et al. Impact of FLT3 internal tandem duplication on the outcome of related and unrelated hematopoietic transplantation for adult acute myeloid leukemia in first remission: a retrospective analysis. J Clin Oncol 2012;30(7):735–41.

17. Whitman SP, Ruppert AS, Radmacher MD, et al. FLT3 D835/I836 mutations are associated with poor disease-free survival and a distinct gene-expression signature among younger adults with de novo cytogenetically normal acute myeloid leukemia lacking FLT3 internal tandem duplications. Blood 2008;111(3):1552–9.

18. Garg M, Nagata Y, Kanojia D, et al. Profiling of somatic mutations in acute myeloid leukemia with FLT3-ITD at diagnosis and relapse. Blood 2015;126(22): 2491–501.

19. Jan M, Snyder TM, Corces-Zimmerman MR, et al. Clonal evolution of preleukemic hematopoietic stem cells precedes human acute myeloid leukemia. Sci Transl Med 2012;4(149):149ra118.

20. Kronke J, Bullinger L, Teleanu V, et al. Clonal evolution in relapsed NPM1-mutated acute myeloid leukemia. Blood 2013;122(1):100–8.

21. Shih LY, Huang CF, Wu JH, et al. Internal tandem duplication of FLT3 in relapsed acute myeloid leukemia: a comparative analysis of bone marrow samples from 108 adult patients at diagnosis and relapse. Blood 2002;100(7):2387–92.

22. Pratz KW, Sato T, Murphy KM, et al. FLT3-mutant allelic burden and clinical status are predictive of response to FLT3 inhibitors in AML. Blood 2010;115(7):1425–32.

23. Smith BD, Levis M, Beran M, et al. Single-agent CEP-701, a novel FLT3 inhibitor, shows biologic and clinical activity in patients with relapsed or refractory acute myeloid leukemia. Blood 2004;103(10):3669–76.

24. Weisberg E, Boulton C, Kelly LM, et al. Inhibition of mutant FLT3 receptors in leukemia cells by the small molecule tyrosine kinase inhibitor PKC412. Cancer cell 2002;1(5):433–43.

25. Stone RM, DeAngelo DJ, Klimek V, et al. Patients with acute myeloid leukemia and an activating mutation in FLT3 respond to a small-molecule FLT3 tyrosine kinase inhibitor, PKC412. Blood 2005;105(1):54–60.

26. Fischer T, Stone RM, Deangelo DJ, et al. Phase IIB trial of oral Midostaurin (PKC412), the FMS-like tyrosine kinase 3 receptor (FLT3) and multi-targeted kinase inhibitor, in patients with acute myeloid leukemia and high-risk myelodysplastic syndrome with either wild-type or mutated FLT3. J Clin Oncol 2010; 28(28):4339–45.

27. Fiedler W, Serve H, Dohner H, et al. A phase 1 study of SU11248 in the treatment of patients with refractory or resistant acute myeloid leukemia (AML) or not amenable to conventional therapy for the disease. Blood 2005;105(3):986–93.

28. Zhang W, Konopleva M, Shi YX, et al. Mutant FLT3: a direct target of sorafenib in acute myelogenous leukemia. J Natl Cancer Inst 2008;100(3):184–98.

29. Crump M, Hedley D, Kamel-Reid S, et al. A randomized phase I clinical and biologic study of two schedules of sorafenib in patients with myelodysplastic syndrome or acute myeloid leukemia: a NCIC (National Cancer Institute of Canada) Clinical Trials Group Study. Leuk Lymphoma 2010;51(2):252–60.

30. Borthakur G, Kantarjian H, Ravandi F, et al. Phase I study of sorafenib in patients with refractory or relapsed acute leukemias. Haematologica 2011;96(1):62–8.

31. Man CH, Fung TK, Ho C, et al. Sorafenib treatment of FLT3-ITD(+) acute myeloid leukemia: favorable initial outcome and mechanisms of subsequent nonresponsiveness associated with the emergence of a D835 mutation. Blood 2012; 119(22):5133–43.

32. Zarrinkar PP, Gunawardane RN, Cramer MD, et al. AC220 is a uniquely potent and selective inhibitor of FLT3 for the treatment of acute myeloid leukemia (AML). Blood 2009;114(14):2984–92.

33. Cortes JE, Kantarjian H, Foran JM, et al. Phase I study of quizartinib administered daily to patients with relapsed or refractory acute myeloid leukemia irrespective of FMS-like tyrosine kinase 3-internal tandem duplication status. J Clin Oncol 2013;31(29):3681–7.

34. Cortes JE, Tallman MS, Schiller G, et al. Results of a phase 2 randomized, open-label, study of lower doses of Quizartinib (AC220; ASP2689) in subjects with FLT3-ITD positive relapsed or refractory acute myeloid leukemia (AML). Paper presented at: American Society of Hematology Annual Meeting. New Orleans, LA, December 7–10, 2013.

35. Schiller GJ, Tallman MS, Goldberg SL, et al. Final results of a randomized phase 2 study showing the clinical benefit of quizartinib (AC220) in patients with FLT3-ITD positive relapsed or refractory acute myeloid leukemia. Paper presented at: American Society of Clinical Oncology Annual Meeting. Chicago, IL, May 30–June 3, 2014.

36. Levis MJ, Martinelli G, Perl AE, et al. The benefit of treatment with quizartinib and subsequent bridging to HSCT for FLT3-ITD(+) patients with AML. Paper presented at: American Society of Clinical Oncology Annual Meeting. Chicago, IL, May 30–June 3, 2014.

37. Smith CC, Wang Q, Chin CS, et al. Validation of ITD mutations in FLT3 as a therapeutic target in human acute myeloid leukaemia. Nature 2012;485(7397):260–3.

38. Zimmerman EI, Turner DC, Buaboonnam J, et al. Crenolanib is active against models of drug-resistant FLT3-ITD-positive acute myeloid leukemia. Blood 2013;122(22):3607–15.

39. Galanis A, Ma H, Rajkhowa T, et al. Crenolanib is a potent inhibitor of FLT3 with activity against resistance-conferring point mutants. Blood 2014;123(1):94–100.

40. Randhawa JK, Kantarjian H, Borthakur G, et al. Results of a Phase II Study of Crenolanib in Relapsed/Refractory Acute Myeloid Leukemia Patients (Pts) with Activating FLT3 Mutations Paper presented at: American Society of Hematology Annual Meeting. San Francisco, CA, December 6–9, 2014.

41. Perl AE, Altman JK, Cortes JE, et al. Final results of the chrysalis trial: a first-in-human phase 1/2 dose-escalation, dose-expansion study of gilteritinib (ASP2215) in patients with relapsed/refractory acute myeloid leukemia (R/R AML). Paper presented at: American Society of Hematology Annual Meeting. San Diego, CA, December 3–6, 2016.

42. Perl AE, Cortes JE, Strickland SA, et al. A phase 3, open-label, randomized study of the FLT3 inhibitor gilteritinib versus salvage chemotherapy in adults with first relapse or primary refractory FLT3 mutation-positive acute myeloid leukemia. Paper presented at: American Society of Clinical Oncology Annual Meeting. Chicago, IL, June 3–7, 2016.

43. Levis M, Ravandi F, Wang ES, et al. Results from a randomized trial of salvage chemotherapy followed by lestaurtinib for patients with FLT3 mutant AML in first relapse. Blood 2011;117(12):3294–301.

44. Fiedler W, Kayser S, Kebenko M, et al. A phase I/II study of sunitinib and intensive chemotherapy in patients over 60 years of age with acute myeloid leukaemia and activating FLT3 mutations. Br J Haematol 2015;169(5):694–700.

45. Ohanian M, Kantajian HM, Borthakur G, et al. Efficacy of a Type I FLT3 Inhibitor, Crenolanib, with Idarubicin and High-Dose Ara-C in Multiply Relapsed/Refractory FLT3+ AML. Paper presented at: American Society of Hematology Annual Meeting. San Diego, CA, December 3–6, 2016.

46. Knapper S, Russell N, Gilkes A, et al. A randomized assessment of adding the kinase inhibitor lestaurtinib to 1st-line chemotherapy for FLT3-mutated AML. Blood 2017;129(9):1143–54.

47. Levis M, Pham R, Smith BD, et al. In vitro studies of a FLT3 inhibitor combined with chemotherapy: sequence of administration is important to achieve synergistic cytotoxic effects. Blood 2004;104(4):1145–50.

48. Ravandi F, Cortes JE, Jones D, et al. Phase I/II study of combination therapy with sorafenib, idarubicin, and cytarabine in younger patients with acute myeloid leukemia. J Clin Oncol 2010;28(11):1856–62.

49. Ravandi F, Arana Yi C, Cortes JE, et al. Final report of phase II study of sorafenib, cytarabine and idarubicin for initial therapy in younger patients with acute myeloid leukemia. Leukemia 2014;28(7):1543–5.

50. Serve H, Krug U, Wagner R, et al. Sorafenib in combination with intensive chemotherapy in elderly patients with acute myeloid leukemia: results from a randomized, placebo-controlled trial. J Clin Oncol 2013;31(25):3110–8.

51. Uy GL, Mandrekar S, Laumann K, et al. Addition of sorafenib to chemotherapy improves the overall surival of older adults with FLT3-ITD mutated acute myeloid leukemia (AML) (Alliance C11001). Paper presented at: American Society of Hematology Annual Meeting. Orlando, FL, December 5–8, 2015.

52. Rollig C, Serve H, Huttmann A, et al. Addition of sorafenib versus placebo to standard therapy in patients aged 60 years or younger with newly diagnosed acute myeloid leukaemia (SORAML): a multicentre, phase 2, randomised controlled trial. Lancet Oncol 2015;16(16):1691–9.

53. Burnett AK, Bowen D, Russel N, et al. AC220 (Quizartinib) can be safely combined with conventional chemotherapy in older patients with newly diagnosed acute myeloid leukaemia: experience from the AML18 Pilot Trial. Paper presented at: American Society of Hematology Annual Meeting. New Orleans, LA, December 7–10, 2013.

54. Erba HP, Levis MJ, Sekeres MA, et al. Phase 3 (P3) study of quizartinib (Q) or placebo (P) with induction (IND) and consolidation chemotherapy (CON) and as maintenance (MN) in patients (pts) with newly diagnosed (NDx) FLT3-ITD–positive acute myeloid leukemia (AML): the QuANTUM-First study. Paper presented at: American Society of Clinical Oncology Annual Meeting. Chicago, IL, June 3–7, 2016.

55. Stone RM, Fischer T, Paquette R, et al. Phase IB study of the FLT3 kinase inhibitor midostaurin with chemotherapy in younger newly diagnosed adult patients with acute myeloid leukemia. Leukemia 2012;26(9):2061–8.

56. Stone RM, Mandrekar S, Sanford BL, et al. The Multi-Kinase Inhibitor Midostaurin (M) Prolongs Survival Compared with Placebo (P) in Combination with Daunorubicin (D)/Cytarabine (C) Induction (ind), High-Dose C Consolidation (consol), and As Maintenance (maint) Therapy in Newly Diagnosed Acute Myeloid Leukemia (AML) Patients (pts) Age 18–60 with FLT3 Mutations (muts): An International Prospective Randomized (rand) P-Controlled Double-Blind Trial (CALGB 10603/RATIFY [Alliance]). Paper presented at: American Society of Hematology Annual Meeting. Orlando, FL, December 5–8, 2015.

57. Schlenk R, Dohner H, Salih H, et al. Midostaurin in combination with intensive induction and as single agent maintenance therapy after consolidation therapy with allogeneic hematopoietic stem cell transplantation or high-dose cytarabine (NCT01477606). Paper presented at: American Society of Hematology Annual Meeting. Orlando, FL, December 5–8, 2015.

58. Wang ES, Stone RM, Tallman MS, et al. Crenolanib, a type I FLT3 TKI, can be safely combined with cytarabine and anthracycline induction chemotherapy and results in high response rates in patients with newly diagnosed FLT3 mutant acute myeloid leukemia (AML). Paper presented at: American Society of Hematology Annual Meeting. San Diego, CA, December 3–6, 2016.

59. Dombret H, Seymour JF, Butrym A, et al. International phase 3 study of azacitidine vs conventional care regimens in older patients with newly diagnosed AML with >30% blasts. Blood 2015;126(3):291–9.

60. Kantarjian HM, Thomas XG, Dmoszynska A, et al. Multicenter, randomized, open-label, phase III trial of decitabine versus patient choice, with physician advice, of either supportive care or low-dose cytarabine for the treatment of older patients with newly diagnosed acute myeloid leukemia. J Clin Oncol 2012;30(21):2670–7.

61. Ravandi F, Alattar ML, Grunwald MR, et al. Phase 2 study of azacytidine plus sorafenib in patients with acute myeloid leukemia and FLT-3 internal tandem duplication mutation. Blood 2013;121(23):4655–62.

62. Sato T, Yang X, Knapper S, et al. FLT3 ligand impedes the efficacy of FLT3 inhibitors in vitro and in vivo. Blood 2011;117(12):3286–93.

63. Yokoyama H, Lundqvist A, Su S, et al. Toxic effects of sorafenib when given early after allogeneic hematopoietic stem cell transplantation. Blood 2010;116(15):2858–9.

64. Chen YB, Li S, Lane AA, et al. Phase I trial of maintenance sorafenib after allogeneic hematopoietic stem cell transplantation for fms-like tyrosine kinase 3 internal tandem duplication acute myeloid leukemia. Biol Blood Marrow Transplant 2014;20(12):2042–8.

65. Sandmaier BM, Khaled SK, Oran B, et al. Results of a Phase 1 Study of Quizartinib (AC220) as maintenance therapy in subjects with acute myeloid leukemia in remission following allogeneic hematopoietic cell transplantation. Paper presented at: American Society of Hematology Annual Meeting. San Francisco, CA, December 6–9, 2014.

Mechanisms of Resistance to FLT3 Inhibitors and the Role of the Bone Marrow Microenvironment

Gabriel Ghiaur, MD, PhD[a],*, Mark Levis, MD, PhD[b]

KEYWORDS

- FLT3 inhibitors • FLT3-ITD • AML • Stem cell niche

KEY POINTS

- Single-agent FLT3 inhibitors can induce remission without cure in FLT3-internal tandem duplication (ITD) acute myeloid leukemia (AML), but to eliminate the last bastion of minimal residual disease (MRD), additional interventions are required.
- Resistance to FLT3 inhibitors may be facilitated by signals from the microenvironment that allow survival of AML cells in the presence of these agents.
- Pharmacokinetics and pharmacodynamics do not always correlate and pharmacodynamics is a better predictor of efficacy when using FLT3 inhibitors.
- FLT3 inhibitors are potent in clearing circulating blasts, yet this does not always translate into similar effects on bone marrow blasts.
- Accumulation of additional mutations in the FLT3-ITD AML clone allows for emergence of clones with cell intrinsic resistance to FLT3 inhibitors.

INTRODUCTION

FLT3-mutated acute myeloid leukemia (AML) represents about one-third of all cases of newly diagnosed AML.[1] Two classes of mutations are frequently found: activation loop or tyrosine kinase domain mutations (TKD; about 5%–10% of patients) and in-frame, internal tandem duplication (ITD; about 23% of patients). Although the prognostic impact of de novo FLT3-TKD mutations is usually minimal, the presence of

G. Ghiaur has nothing to disclose. M. Levis receives research funding from Novartis and Astellas. M. Levis serves as a consultant for Novartis, Daiichi-Sankyo, Astellas, and Arog.
[a] Adult Leukemia Program, Division of Hematological Malignancies, Sidney Kimmel Comprehensive Cancer Center, Johns Hopkins University, 1650 Orleans Street CRB I, Room 243, Baltimore, MD 21287, USA; [b] Adult Leukemia Program, Division of Hematological Malignancies, Sidney Kimmel Comprehensive Cancer Center, Johns Hopkins University, 1650 Orleans Street CRB I, Room 2M44, Baltimore, MD 21287, USA
* Corresponding author.
E-mail address: gghiaur1@jhmi.edu

Hematol Oncol Clin N Am 31 (2017) 681–692
http://dx.doi.org/10.1016/j.hoc.2017.04.005
0889-8588/17/© 2017 Elsevier Inc. All rights reserved.

hemonc.theclinics.com

FLT3-ITD mutations confers a poor prognosis in AML[2–4] and the frequency of the mutated allele (allelic ratio)[4] as well as the length of the tandem repeat (ITD length) correlate with worse outcomes.[5]

FLT3 is a class III receptor tyrosine kinase that dimerizes upon ligand binding and undergoes autophosphorylation to initiate multiple intracellular signaling programs.[6] These pathways, including PI3K/AKT, Jak/STAT, and Ras/MAPK, transduce signals resulting in survival and proliferation of target cells (**Fig. 1**).

During normal hematopoiesis, FLT3 is expressed in early progenitor cells and the receptor is downregulated while cells differentiate down the myeloid lineage. Patients with FLT3-mutated AML not only have constitutively active signaling but, given the lack of differentiation, these AML blasts continue to express high levels of this mutated protein in addition to the wild-type FLT3 receptor.[7]

This sustained survival and proliferation signal is the hallmark of FLT3-mutated AML. The clinical presentation of these patients is dominated by hyperleukocytosis, myeloblastic/monoblastic differentiation and usually de novo (as opposed to secondary) AML. Compared with other poor prognostic factors in AML, the presence of an FLT3-ITD mutation does not have a major impact on achieving remission after induction chemotherapy, but the remission is characteristically short lived and relapse often occurs during cycles of consolidation (sometimes while an allogeneic donor search is underway). There is a consensus that prompt blood or marrow transplantation in first remission can improve the outcome in this disease even in the absence of FLT3 inhibitors. Nevertheless, the high rate of relapse even posttransplantation makes this approach alone suboptimal.

In the setting of relapsed disease, the FLT3-ITD mutation is often present at a high allelic ratio,[8] and the mutated receptor in the malignant clone renders this disease resistant to chemotherapy. At this stage, the blasts are addicted to signaling downstream of this RTK and, thus, sensitive to FLT3 inhibitors. Thus, the clinical development of small molecule inhibitors that target mutant FLT3 is an active area of research. More than 60 clinical trials are either open or completed testing different FLT3 inhibitors as single agents or in combination with other therapeutic approaches in AML (available at: clinicaltrials.gov). Full updates on the clinical development of these strategies can be found in this issue (See Jacqueline S. Garcia and Richard M. Stone's article, "The Development of FLT3 Inhibitors in Acute Myeloid Leukemia," in this issue). Herein, we focus our attention on mechanisms of resistance to FLT3 inhibitors and strategies to overcome such resistance and achieve cure in FLT3-mutated AML.

MECHANISMS THAT ALLOW SURVIVAL OF FLT3-MUTATED ACUTE MYELOID LEUKEMIA CELLS DURING TREATMENT WITH FLT3 INHIBITORS

Wisdom gathered from more than 7 decades of antimicrobial use to treat infections tells us that resistance to treatment is either acquired via genetic adaptation or relies on clones already present that are selected under survival pressure. In AML, resistance to chemotherapy can take either one of these two forms. Elegant genetic studies have shown that AML at diagnosis is a polyclonal disease, whereas relapsed AML is usually more oligoclonal.[9] Most of the time, the relapsed clone can be retrospectively found at presentation but at much lower frequency. This pattern seems to be the case with FLT3-mutated AML relapsing after induction chemotherapy. Most of the initial malignant subclones are sensitive to treatment and the patient achieves a clean complete remission. Nevertheless, some clones survive chemotherapy and are responsible for disease relapse. At relapse, the mutant allelic ratio is often higher than what was seen at diagnosis.

In contrast, it is probable that the development of resistance to FLT3 inhibitors is at least in part dependent on some genetic or epigenetic events. For these genetic and epigenetic events to take place, some FLT3 mutated cells will need to have survived the initial treatment.

Initial studies using FLT3 inhibitors demonstrated clearance of circulating FLT3-ITD blasts, but there was little to no effect on bone marrow blasts.[10] More potent and selective FLT3 inhibitors are effective at differentiating most bone marrow blasts,[11] but since these drugs cannot eliminate minimal residual disease as single agents, some leukemia cells, perhaps residing in the stem cell niche, must survive the treatment with the inhibitor.

Potential mechanism that contribute to survival of leukemia blasts in the stem cell niche during treatment with FLT3 inhibitors fall into two categories: a) signaling mechanisms that bypass the effective inhibition of FLT3 receptor and b) suboptimal pharmacokinetics and phamacodynamics in the stem cell niche.

Bypassing the FLT3 Receptor

This early evidence pointed toward stromal mediated mechanisms of survival. To this end, coculture of FLT3-ITD AML cells with bone marrow mesenchymal stroma also protects the blasts from quizartinib[12] as well as Fl-700.[13] In these settings, soluble as well as membrane-bound cytokines that seem to play a major role include CXCL12, angiopoietins, as well as vascular endothelial growth factor/epidermal growth factor/insulin-like growth factor and granulocyte colony stimulating factor/granulocyte macrophage colony stimulating factor/tumor necrosis factor.[12,13] Similarly, patients with FLT3-ITD AML treated with quizartinib develop high levels of stromal-derived fibroblast growth factor 2 in bone marrow mesenchymal cells. Pathways downstream of fibroblast growth factor receptor 1 maintain active RAS/MAPK signaling in FLT3-ITD blasts treated with quizartinib.[14] Most patients with FLT3-ITD continue to have a wild-type allele of FLT3. This receptor is rather resistant to FLT3 inhibitors but sensitive to FLT3 ligand. Because high levels of FLT3 ligand are found in the bone marrow microenvironment during induction therapy, ligand-induced activation of the wild-type FLT3–MAPK pathway may provide survival signals to leukemic blasts, even in the presence of effective TKI treatment.[14,15]

Potent FLT3-ITD inhibition results in apoptosis of AML blasts in the absence of stroma. The presence of bone marrow mesenchymal stroma rescues the blasts from apoptosis through extracellular receptor kinase (ERK)-mediated signaling but not STAT5.[12] In this context, inhibition of FLT3-ITD induces G1 arrest, possibly via downregulation of cyclin D2/cyclin D3 and subsequent dephosphorylation of Rb.[16] Individual FLT3 inhibitors may have differential effects, for instance, contact with niche cells expand FLT3-ITD blasts treated with SU5615 but not sorafenib.[17]

Suboptimal Pharmacokinetics and Pharmacodynamics

Complete and sustained inhibition of FLT3-ITD is paramount for the successful elimination of the malignant clone. Initial studies with midostaurin clearly demonstrated the impact of hepatic drug metabolism and CYP3A4 activity in particular of this drug plasma pharmacokinetics. More so, pharmacodynamic studies have shown wide variations between systemic concentrations and plasma inhibitory activity of various TKIs, likely owing to unique protein binding affinities of specific drugs. Pharmacodynamic-directed dose escalation clinical studies have mitigated these limitations for the most part and resulted in improved efficacy in clearing not only circulating blasts, but also most bone marrow disease. Recent work proposes the existence of unique niches in the bone marrow, some of which are true biochemical sanctuaries where local drug levels may be significantly different from systemic plasma drug levels.[18] To this end, bone marrow mesenchymal stroma expresses similar levels of drug metabolizing enzymes compared with

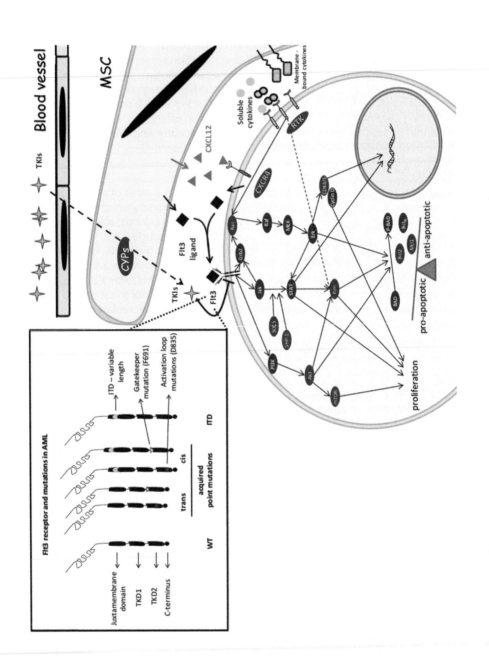

hepatocytes. They are able to metabolize CYP3A4 substrates, creating potential biochemical spaces where FLT3 inhibitors achieve levels inadequate for potent inhibition of FLT3-ITD.

EMERGENCE OF RESISTANCE

Initially, survival in the setting of TKI therapy probably happens in remote and unique niches within the bone marrow, and thus relies on the presence of a minute population of leukemia stem cells. The emergence of clinical resistance is most likely preceded by cell intrinsic events that allow the new clone to leave the "nest" and dominate the organism. Accumulating knowledge from studying the emergence of resistance to imatinib in chronic myelogenous leukemia points toward two types of resistance: (a) mutation in the target receptor or (b) activation of alternative pathways that bypass the mutant receptor.

Mutations in the Target Receptor

A variety of FLT3 mutations that could confer resistance to FLT3 inhibitors have been predicted based on in vitro models of resistance. Some of these predicted mutations have been confirmed in patients relapsing with FLT3 mutated disease during treatment with FLT3 inhibitors.

Most FLT3 inhibitors are active against FLT3-ITD, but have limited activity against TKD mutants. Even though a TKD mutation may have only minimal prognostic value when present at diagnosis, the appearance of point mutations in the FLT3 receptor is a major mechanism of resistance to FLT3 inhibitors (see **Fig. 1**). These point mutant can develop either in cis or in trans and newer FLT3 inhibitors have various degrees of activity against individual mutants.[19]

It is important to recognize that, depending on the domain used to bind the receptor, FLT3 inhibitors can be segregated in two classes: type I inhibitors, like CEP-701, PKC-412, and crenolanib, bind to the "gatekeeper" domain adjacent to the activation loop or the ATP-binding domain; type II inhibitors, like sorafenib, quizartinib, and MLN518, directly bind the ATP-binding domain. As expected, point mutants conferring resistance to one TKI show cross-resistance within the class. To this end, patients with FLT3-ITD that relapse while treated with quizartinib, if they are found to have point mutations in the activation loop (most frequent D835) or "gatekeeping" domain (ie, F691), usually show resistance to sorafenib, another type II TKI. Interestingly, these cells remain sensitive to type I TKIs such as PKC412 and crenolanib.[20] Similarly, some TKIs, like the type I inhibitor TTT-3002, demonstrate preclinical potential to target both type of mutations.[21]

Activation of Alternative Signaling Pathways

Although intensively studied, the accumulation of additional mutations in the FLT3 receptor represents a minority of cases developing resistance to FLT3 inhibitors. In a small study following 60 patients with FLT3-ITD alone treated with single-agent TKI,

---

Fig. 1. FLT3 signaling and mechanisms of resistance to FLT3 inhibitors. Wild-type (WT) as well as FLT3-mutated receptor signal via Jak/STAT, PI3K/Akt and Ras/MAPK to provide anti-apoptotic as well as proliferative signaling to the leukemic blasts. Mechanisms that maintain these pathways active in the presence of FLT3 inhibitors create the conditions for the development of resistance. Combining FLT3 inhibitors with inhibitors of these pathways hold the promise of preventing development of resistance. Potential targets are highlighted in red. Point mutations in the FLT3 receptor are detailed in the rectangular insert. AML, acute myeloid leukemia; ITD, internal tandem duplication; MSC, mesenchymal stem cells; TKIs, tyrosine kinase inhibitors.

two-thirds of patients progressed on FLT3 inhibitor treatment even though they showed no additional mutations in FLT3 wild-type allele or FLT3-ITD. Only 22% of patients acquired additional mutations, all of them D835 or I836.[22] Thus, alternative mechanisms of resistance, independent of FLT3 receptor, must be playing a major role and recent studies have uncovered some of these pathways.

Generally, these pathways either provide survival signals independent of FLT3-ITD or they change the transcriptional factor network of the leukemic cell to a state where FLT3 signaling can be replaced by activation of other RTKs.

As mentioned, FLT3-ITD can activate signaling cascades downstream of JAK/STAT, PI3K/AKT, and MAPK pathways. Because blasts become addicted to this constitutively active signaling, FLT3 inhibitors induce rapid apoptosis. Although microenvironmental factors may rescue these cells in the stem cell niche (see above), the development of cell intrinsic mechanisms that can protect these cells from apoptosis coincide with development of resistance to TKIs. FLT3-ITD changes the balance between antiapoptotic proteins, such as Bcl2/Bcl$_{XL}$, and proapoptotic Bcl-2-associated death promoter (BAD) (**Fig. 1**). Sustained activation of phospho-STAT5 by FLT3-ITD signaling, for instance, activates Pim kinases that, in turn, by phosphorylating BAD, sequesters these proteins in the cytoplasm and allows antiapoptotic activities of Bcl2 and Bcl$_{XL}$.[23,24] Inhibition of FLT3-ITD results in rapid loss of phospho-STAT5 and downregulation of Pim-1.[23] Cells resistant to FLT3 inhibitors show sustained activity of Pim-1[23] or Pim-2[25,26] and high levels of phospho-BAD and, thus, protection from apoptosis. Thus, combined inhibitions of FLT3-ITD and Pim1[27] or Pim-2[26] are synergistic in inducing apoptosis in mutant blasts. Similarly, high levels of Bcl2 can also confer resistance to FLT3 inhibitors. In these settings, the use of Bcl2 inhibitors such as ABT-737[28] rescues FLT3 inhibitor–induced apoptosis of mutated cells. Interestingly, FLT3-ITD/TKD mutants that show sustained activation of phospho-STAT5 also exhibit elevated levels of antiapoptotic signals mediated by Bcl$_{XL}$.[29] In these models, inhibition of the mammalian target of rapamycin (mTOR) pathway can rescue the sensitivity of these cells to both FLT3 inhibitors and anthracyclines.[29] Similarly, cells resistant to sorafenib continue to have an active mTOR/PI3K/Akt pathway even in the presence of effective FLT3 inhibition,[30,31] and mTOR inhibitors can resensitize the blasts to TKI.[30] Some FLT3-ITD point mutations (D627 E) can induce expression of Mcl-1 (a Bcl-2 family member) independent of kinase activity via a conformational change that favors Grb-2 docking.[32] Because Mcl-1, in addition to its antiapoptotic roles, also impacts mitochondrial morphology and function,[33] it is not surprising that sorafenib resistant cells adopt an abnormal mitochondrial respiratory chain and rely mostly on glycolysis for their energy demands.[34] Thus, glycolytic inhibitors like 2-deoxyglucose can resensitize cells to sorafenib.[34] Of note, a major limitation to a predominantly glycolytic metabolism is a sustained decrease in intracellular pH. Consistent with this concept, FLT3-ITD cells developing resistance to sorafenib also upregulated tescalcin, a type I Na/H exchange channel. Downregulation of this protein or inhibition via amiloride reduced leukemia initiation in xenograft models of sorafenib-resistant FLT3-ITD AML.[35]

Maintaining an active MAPK/ERK pathway either by expression of constitutively Axl-1[36] or acquiring activating mutations in NRAS[31] has also been shown to be potential mechanisms of resistance to FLT3 inhibitors.

Epigenetic events, particularly methylation of target genes, have been proposed as potential mechanisms of resistance to FLT3 inhibitors. To this end, methylation of SHP-1[37] and silencing of SOCS proteins[38] both negative regulators of JAK/STAT pathway have been implicated in resistance to FLT3-inhibitors. Treatment with DNMT inhibitors not only rescues expression of these proteins but also resensitizes the cells to the TKI.[37]

STRATEGIES TO PREVENT THE DEVELOPMENT OF RESISTANCE OR TO SENSITIZE CELLS TO FLT3 INHIBITORS

Initial agents used to treat patients with FLT3-ITD had broader activity against multiple receptor tyrosine kinases but also less-than-ideal pharmacologic properties. Recently developed inhibitors are more specific and very potent. More targeted agents have fewer side effects and, thus, higher doses can be used. In contrast, agents that inhibit multiple RTKs may prevent emergence of resistance via these mechanisms. Plasma inhibitory assay–directed studies have overcome some of the primary failure seen with single-agent FLT3-inhibitors and helped to optimize the dosage for newer drugs.

Given the type of secondary mutations that can arise in the FLT3 receptor during treatment with FLT3 inhibitors, it was suggested that switching to a different class of inhibitor may prove beneficial in these patients. Ponatinib, for instance, is effective against gate keeper mutations (F691) that arise during treatment with quizartinib, but not against activation loop mutations (D835).[39] In the same study, SAR302503, a dual Jak2/FLT3 inhibitor, was highly effective in vitro against both types of mutants. On the same note, crenolanib, a type I inhibitor is effective against FLT3-ITD–expressing cells that became resistant to sorafenib via accumulation of mutations in both activation loop[40,41] and gate keeper mutations.[41] Similarly, G-749, a FLT3 inhibitor active against multiple activation loop as well as gate keeper mutations, has shown great efficiency in xenograft models of FLT3-ITD AML that would be otherwise resistant to quizartinib or PKC412.[42]

Although single-agent FLT3 inhibitors can induce remission, the complete eradication of disease relies on combination therapy. There are a number of preclinical studies that investigate the efficiency of concomitant targeting of FLT3 signaling as well as pathways implicated in resistance. For instance, targeting the ERK/MAPK pathway either by inhibition of upstream RTK such as Axl1,[36] inhibition of MEK,[43] MERTK,[44] or NRas[31] with small molecules, showed promising activity in preclinical models, including xenografts of FLT3-ITD AML. This approach of multi kinase inhibition can likely bypass the stromal protection against FLT3 inhibitors and decrease emergence of resistance.[12] To this end, a promising strategy is targeting Pim kinases (known to be upregulated in response to cytokines produced by the mesenchymal stroma). The combination of Pim1/Pim2 inhibitors with FLT3 inhibitors is active against FLT3-ITD AML in preclinical models.[26] Additionally, agents that target antiapoptotic mechanisms important in FLT3-ITD signaling have shown activity in AML blasts in combination with FLT3 inhibitors. To this end, a dual inhibitor of Akt/FLT3-ITD, A674563, can overcome FLT3 ligand-induced drug resistance in vitro and in xenograft models.[45] Similarly, mTOR inhibition can sensitize cells to FLT3 inhibition,[29] likely via targeting signaling downstream of PI3K.[30] An alternative approach that showed preclinical activity is to directly target Bcl2. In this regard, ABT-737 has shown synergistic effects with FLT3 inhibitors against FLT3-ITD AML.[46] Corroborated with preliminary data coming from clinical studies using Bcl2 inhibitors agents in other AML subtypes, it may be of interest to study the effects of FLT3 inhibitors in combination with Bcl2 inhibitors in clinical studies.

As mentioned, a potential mechanism that is associated with resistance to FLT3 inhibitors relies on CDK4/6 activity and their impact on either cyclin D2/cyclin D3 or direct transcriptional activation of FLT3 and Pim kinases. Targeting this mechanism with either the dual CDK4/FLT3-ITD inhibitor, AMG925[47,48] or by adding palbociclib,[49] a CDK6 inhibitor, showed promise to sensitize resistant cells to FLT3 inhibitors.

Because the survival of FLT3-ITD leukemia cells depends on absolute levels of FLT3-ITD, decreasing oncoprotein stability using Hsp90 inhibitors[50] or activating autophagy via proteasome inhibitors like bortezomib[51] can also resensitize resistant FLT3-ITD AML cells to TKI. Last, in a small case series, concomitant treatment with cyclosporine benefitted patients with FLT3-ITD AML who were being treated with FLT3 inhibitors, perhaps via inhibition of NFATc1.[52] This mechanism of sensitization will need to be compared in larger patient studies before definitive conclusions can be drawn.

OUR APPROACH TO RESISTANT FLT3-INTERNAL TANDEM DUPLICATION ACUTE MYELOID LEUKEMIA

Despite all the potentially available strategies to overcome resistance to TKIs, the treatment of patients with FLT3-ITD AML relapsing while on FLT3 inhibitors remains a major clinical challenge. Our current strategy relies on enrollment in a clinical trial if available. If not available, one of the most promising approaches in our clinic is the use of the combination of FLT3 inhibitors (eg, sorafenib) with hypomethylating agents. We prefer 5-aza-citidine,[53,54] but other groups have shown similar results with decitabine. In patients receiving sorafenib and 5-azacitidine, the leukemia undergoes differentiation. There is a gradual decrease of bone marrow blasts to the point where, after 3 cycles, 40% to 50% of these patients have achieved a morphologic remission. To date, it remains unclear how 5-azacitidine or decitabine sensitizes FLT3-ITD cells to TKI, but mechanisms may include reexpression of methylated genes such as SOCS1, SOCS2, SOCS3,[38] or SHP-1,[37] or even tumor debulking without the associated increased in FLT3 ligand seen with classical chemotherapy.[54] Last, it was suggested that DNMT inhibitors may sensitize cells to FLT3 inhibitors via their prodifferentiation effects.[53] Treatment with 5-azacitidine for instance, decreases total FLT3-ITD protein levels as cells differentiate and, thus, make them more sensitive to a FLT3 inhibitor. To this end, differentiation agents such as homoharringtonine[55] or all-trans retinoic acid[56] have been shown to synergize with FLT3 inhibitors in inducing apoptosis in FLT3-mutated AML. To what extent these are viable approaches to not only control the bulk of the tumor, but also to eliminate MRD and prevent resistance remains to be tested in clinical studies. Moreover, recent evidence suggests that some bone marrow niches may inactivate retinoids and thus, protect malignant cells from differentiation.[57–59]

For this reason, patients with FLT3-ITD that achieve remission after treatment with FLT3 inhibitor plus 5-azacitidine still go on to receive allogeneic transplantation in our center. In addition, it is our experience that treatment with a FLT3 inhibitor posttransplant helps to maintain disease burden to undetectable levels. This may be mediated via both a direct effect on the leukemia clone as well as potential immune modulatory effect of FLT3 inhibitors. Nevertheless, many of these patients do experience various degrees of graft versus host symptoms. To what extent this approach will translate into a viable clinical option is currently being investigated in a Blood and Marrow Clinical Trials Network (BMT CTN) clinical trial.

REFERENCES

1. Levis M, Small D. FLT3: ITDoes matter in leukemia. Leukemia 2003;17(9): 1738–52.
2. Kottaridis PD, Gale RE, Langabeer SE, et al. Studies of FLT3 mutations in paired presentation and relapse samples from patients with acute myeloid leukemia: implications for the role of FLT3 mutations in leukemogenesis, minimal residual disease detection, and possible therapy with FLT3 inhibitors. Blood 2002;100(7):2393–8.
3. Schnittger S, Schoch C, Dugas M, et al. Analysis of FLT3 length mutations in 1003 patients with acute myeloid leukemia: correlation to cytogenetics, FAB subtype,

and prognosis in the AMLCG study and usefulness as a marker for the detection of minimal residual disease. Blood 2002;100(1):59–66.

4. Thiede C, Steudel C, Mohr B, et al. Analysis of FLT3-activating mutations in 979 patients with acute myelogenous leukemia: association with FAB subtypes and identification of subgroups with poor prognosis. Blood 2002;99(12):4326–35.

5. Kayser S, Schlenk RF, Londono MC, et al. Insertion of FLT3 internal tandem duplication in the tyrosine kinase domain-1 is associated with resistance to chemotherapy and inferior outcome. Blood 2009;114(12):2386–92.

6. Rosnet O, Buhring HJ, deLapeyriere O, et al. Expression and signal transduction of the FLT3 tyrosine kinase receptor. Acta Haematol 1996;95(3–4):218–23.

7. Carow CE, Levenstein M, Kaufmann SH, et al. Expression of the hematopoietic growth factor receptor FLT3 (STK-1/Flk2) in human leukemias. Blood 1996; 87(3):1089–96.

8. Pratz KW, Sato T, Murphy KM, et al. FLT3-mutant allelic burden and clinical status are predictive of response to FLT3 inhibitors in AML. Blood 2010;115(7):1425–32.

9. Ding L, Ley TJ, Larson DE, et al. Clonal evolution in relapsed acute myeloid leukaemia revealed by whole-genome sequencing. Nature 2012;481(7382): 506–10.

10. Smith BD, Levis M, Beran M, et al. Single-agent CEP-701, a novel FLT3 inhibitor, shows biologic and clinical activity in patients with relapsed or refractory acute myeloid leukemia. Blood 2004;103(10):3669–76.

11. Sexauer A, Perl A, Yang X, et al. Terminal myeloid differentiation in vivo is induced by FLT3 inhibition in FLT3/ITD AML. Blood 2012;120(20):4205–14.

12. Yang X, Sexauer A, Levis M. Bone marrow stroma-mediated resistance to FLT3 inhibitors in FLT3-ITD AML is mediated by persistent activation of extracellular regulated kinase. Br J Haematol 2014;164(1):61–72.

13. Kojima K, McQueen T, Chen Y, et al. p53 activation of mesenchymal stromal cells partially abrogates microenvironment-mediated resistance to FLT3 inhibition in AML through HIF-1alpha-mediated down-regulation of CXCL12. Blood 2011; 118(16):4431–9.

14. Traer E, Martinez J, Javidi-Sharifi N, et al. FGF2 from marrow microenvironment promotes resistance to FLT3 inhibitors in acute myeloid leukemia. Cancer Res 2016;76(22):6471–82.

15. Chen F, Ishikawa Y, Akashi A, et al. Co-expression of wild-type FLT3 attenuates the inhibitory effect of FLT3 inhibitor on FLT3 mutated leukemia cells. Oncotarget 2016;7(30):47018–32.

16. Wang L, Wang J, Blaser BW, et al. Pharmacologic inhibition of CDK4/6: mechanistic evidence for selective activity or acquired resistance in acute myeloid leukemia. Blood 2007;110(6):2075–83.

17. Parmar A, Marz S, Rushton S, et al. Stromal niche cells protect early leukemic FLT3-ITD+ progenitor cells against first-generation FLT3 tyrosine kinase inhibitors. Cancer Res 2011;71(13):4696–706.

18. Alonso S, Su M, Jones JW, et al. Human bone marrow niche chemoprotection mediated by cytochrome P450 enzymes. Oncotarget 2015;6(17):14905–12.

19. Grundler R, Thiede C, Miething C, et al. Sensitivity toward tyrosine kinase inhibitors varies between different activating mutations of the FLT3 receptor. Blood 2003;102(2):646–51.

20. Zhang W, Gao C, Konopleva M, et al. Reversal of acquired drug resistance in FLT3-mutated acute myeloid leukemia cells via distinct drug combination strategies. Clin Cancer Res 2014;20(9):2363–74.

21. Ma HS, Nguyen B, Duffield AS, et al. FLT3 kinase inhibitor TTT-3002 overcomes both activating and drug resistance mutations in FLT3 in acute myeloid leukemia. Cancer Res 2014;74(18):5206–17.

22. Alvarado Y, Kantarjian HM, Luthra R, et al. Treatment with FLT3 inhibitor in patients with FLT3-mutated acute myeloid leukemia is associated with development of secondary FLT3-tyrosine kinase domain mutations. Cancer 2014;120(14): 2142–9.

23. Kim KT, Baird K, Ahn JY, et al. Pim-1 is up-regulated by constitutively activated FLT3 and plays a role in FLT3-mediated cell survival. Blood 2005;105(4):1759–67.

24. Kim KT, Levis M, Small D. Constitutively activated FLT3 phosphorylates BAD partially through pim-1. Br J Haematol 2006;134(5):500–9.

25. Adam M, Pogacic V, Bendit M, et al. Targeting PIM kinases impairs survival of hematopoietic cells transformed by kinase inhibitor-sensitive and kinase inhibitor-resistant forms of Fms-like tyrosine kinase 3 and BCR/ABL. Cancer Res 2006; 66(7):3828–35.

26. Green AS, Maciel TT, Hospital MA, et al. Pim kinases modulate resistance to FLT3 tyrosine kinase inhibitors in FLT3-ITD acute myeloid leukemia. Sci Adv 2015;1(8): e1500221.

27. Fathi AT, Arowojolu O, Swinnen I, et al. A potential therapeutic target for FLT3-ITD AML: PIM1 kinase. Leuk Res 2012;36(2):224–31.

28. Kohl TM, Hellinger C, Ahmed F, et al. BH3 mimetic ABT-737 neutralizes resistance to FLT3 inhibitor treatment mediated by FLT3-independent expression of BCL2 in primary AML blasts. Leukemia 2007;21(8):1763–72.

29. Bagrintseva K, Geisenhof S, Kern R, et al. FLT3-ITD-TKD dual mutants associated with AML confer resistance to FLT3 PTK inhibitors and cytotoxic agents by overexpression of Bcl-x(L). Blood 2005;105(9):3679–85.

30. Lindblad O, Cordero E, Puissant A, et al. Aberrant activation of the PI3K/mTOR pathway promotes resistance to sorafenib in AML. Oncogene 2016;35(39): 5119–31.

31. Piloto O, Wright M, Brown P, et al. Prolonged exposure to FLT3 inhibitors leads to resistance via activation of parallel signaling pathways. Blood 2007;109(4): 1643–52.

32. Breitenbuecher F, Markova B, Kasper S, et al. A novel molecular mechanism of primary resistance to FLT3-kinase inhibitors in AML. Blood 2009;113(17): 4063–73.

33. Perciavalle RM, Stewart DP, Koss B, et al. Anti-apoptotic MCL-1 localizes to the mitochondrial matrix and couples mitochondrial fusion to respiration. Nat Cell Biol 2012;14(6):575–83.

34. Huang A, Ju HQ, Liu K, et al. Metabolic alterations and drug sensitivity of tyrosine kinase inhibitor resistant leukemia cells with a FLT3/ITD mutation. Cancer Lett 2016;377(2):149–57.

35. Man CH, Lam SS, Sun MK, et al. A novel tescalcin-sodium/hydrogen exchange axis underlying sorafenib resistance in FLT3-ITD+ AML. Blood 2014;123(16): 2530–9.

36. Park IK, Mundy-Bosse B, Whitman SP, et al. Receptor tyrosine kinase Axl is required for resistance of leukemic cells to FLT3-targeted therapy in acute myeloid leukemia. Leukemia 2015;29(12):2382–9.

37. Al-Jamal HA, Mat Jusoh SA, Hassan R, et al. Enhancing SHP-1 expression with 5-azacytidine may inhibit STAT3 activation and confer sensitivity in lestaurtinib (CEP-701)-resistant FLT3-ITD positive acute myeloid leukemia. BMC Cancer 2015;15:869.

38. Zhou J, Bi C, Janakakumara JV, et al. Enhanced activation of STAT pathways and overexpression of survivin confer resistance to FLT3 inhibitors and could be therapeutic targets in AML. Blood 2009;113(17):4052–62.

39. Kesarwani M, Huber E, Azam M. Overcoming AC220 resistance of FLT3-ITD by SAR302503. Blood Cancer J 2013;3:e138.

40. Galanis A, Ma H, Rajkhowa T, et al. Crenolanib is a potent inhibitor of FLT3 with activity against resistance-conferring point mutants. Blood 2014;123(1):94–100.

41. Zimmerman EI, Turner DC, Buaboonnam J, et al. Crenolanib is active against models of drug-resistant FLT3-ITD-positive acute myeloid leukemia. Blood 2013;122(22):3607–15.

42. Lee HK, Kim HW, Lee IY, et al. G-749, a novel FLT3 kinase inhibitor, can overcome drug resistance for the treatment of acute myeloid leukemia. Blood 2014;123(14):2209–19.

43. Zhang W, Borthakur G, Gao C, et al. The dual MEK/FLT3 inhibitor E6201 exerts cytotoxic activity against acute myeloid leukemia cells harboring resistance-conferring FLT3 mutations. Cancer Res 2016;76(6):1528–37.

44. Minson KA, Smith CC, DeRyckere D, et al. The MERTK/FLT3 inhibitor MRX-2843 overcomes resistance-conferring FLT3 mutations in acute myeloid leukemia. JCI Insight 2016;1(3):e85630.

45. Wang A, Wu H, Chen C, et al. Dual inhibition of AKT/FLT3-ITD by A674563 overcomes FLT3 ligand-induced drug resistance in FLT3-ITD positive AML. Oncotarget 2016;7(20):29131–42.

46. Kohl TM, Hellinger C, Ahmed F, et al. BH3 mimetic ABT-737 neutralizes resistance to FLT3 inhibitor treatment mediated by FLT3-independent expression of BCL2 in primary AML blasts. Leukemia 2007;21(8):1763–72.

47. Keegan K, Li C, Li Z, et al. Preclinical evaluation of AMG 925, a FLT3/CDK4 dual kinase inhibitor for treating acute myeloid leukemia. Mol Cancer Ther 2014;13(4):880–9.

48. Li C, Liu L, Liang L, et al. AMG 925 is a dual FLT3/CDK4 inhibitor with the potential to overcome FLT3 inhibitor resistance in acute myeloid leukemia. Mol Cancer Ther 2015;14(2):375–83.

49. Uras IZ, Walter GJ, Scheicher R, et al. Palbociclib treatment of FLT3-ITD+ AML cells uncovers a kinase-dependent transcriptional regulation of FLT3 and PIM1 by CDK6. Blood 2016;127(23):2890–902.

50. Yu C, Kancha RK, Duyster J. Targeting oncoprotein stability overcomes drug resistance caused by FLT3 kinase domain mutations. PLoS one 2014;9(5):e97116.

51. Larrue C, Saland E, Boutzen H, et al. Proteasome inhibitors induce FLT3-ITD degradation through autophagy in AML cells. Blood 2016;127(7):882–92.

52. Metzelder SK, Michel C, von Bonin M, et al. NFATc1 as a therapeutic target in FLT3-ITD-positive AML. Leukemia 2015;29(7):1470–7.

53. Chang E, Ganguly S, Rajkhowa T, et al. The combination of FLT3 and DNA methyltransferase inhibition is synergistically cytotoxic to FLT3/ITD acute myeloid leukemia cells. Leukemia 2016;30(5):1025–32.

54. Ravandi F, Alattar ML, Grunwald MR, et al. Phase 2 study of azacytidine plus sorafenib in patients with acute myeloid leukemia and FLT-3 internal tandem duplication mutation. Blood 2013;121(23):4655–62.

55. Xu G, Mao L, Liu H, et al. Sorafenib in combination with low-dose-homoharringtonine as a salvage therapy in primary refractory FLT3-ITD-positive AML: a case report and review of literature. Int J Clin Exp Med 2015;8(11):19891–4.

56. Ma HS, Greenblatt SM, Shirley CM, et al. All-trans retinoic acid synergizes with FLT3 inhibition to eliminate FLT3/ITD+ leukemia stem cells in vitro and in vivo. Blood 2016;127(23):2867–78.

57. Alonso S, Hernandez D, Chang YT, et al. Hedgehog and retinoid signaling alters multiple myeloma microenvironment and generates bortezomib resistance. J Clin Invest 2016;126(12):4460–8.

58. Ghiaur G, Yegnasubramanian S, Perkins B, et al. Regulation of human hematopoietic stem cell self-renewal by the microenvironment's control of retinoic acid signaling. Proc Natl Acad Sci U S A 2013;110(40):16121–6.

59. Su M, Alonso S, Jones JW, et al. All-trans retinoic acid activity in acute myeloid leukemia: role of cytochrome P450 enzyme expression by the microenvironment. PLoS one 2015;10(6):e0127790.

Kinase Inhibitor Screening in Myeloid Malignancies

Jeffrey W. Tyner, PhD

KEYWORDS

- Functional screening • Small-molecule inhibitors • Personalized medicine
- Precision medicine • Functional genomics • Chronic neutrophilic leukemia
- Atypical CML

KEY POINTS

- Kinases are common drug targets in myeloid malignancies.
- Kinase dysregulation occurs through a diversity of known and unknown mechanisms.
- Functional screening with kinase inhibitors can foster identification of important kinase targets in myeloid leukemia patient subsets.
- Combining functional screening with genomic data can accelerate understanding of the mechanistic etiology of kinase pathway dependence.

INTRODUCTION

Cancer therapy that is targeted to causative genetic abnormalities has achieved dramatic clinical outcomes in certain malignancy subsets.[1–4] Broad application of this strategy requires a precision medicine approach in which key targets of pathway dysregulation can be rapidly assigned to specific therapeutics in individual patients. The tyrosine kinase gene family, in particular, has played a prominent role as novel targets for cancer therapy over the past several decades.

KINASES AS GENE TARGETS IN MYELOID MALIGNANCY

There are several reasons that kinases and kinase inhibitors have been so broadly explored as cancer therapeutics:

1. Tyrosine kinases play an integral role in numerous cellular processes as diverse as proliferation, apoptosis, differentiation, and cell motililty[5,6]; therefore, dysregulation of tyrosine kinase pathways is likely to contribute to the oncogenic process.
2. There are many examples of specific kinases, both mutated and wild type, that have been directly implicated in the pathogenesis of numerous cancer subsets.[7]

Department of Cell, Developmental and Cancer Biology, Knight Cancer Institute, Oregon Health and Science University, OHSU BRB 511, Mailcode L592, 3181 Southwest Sam Jackson Park Road, Portland, OR 97239, USA
E-mail address: tynerj@ohsu.edu

Hematol Oncol Clin N Am 31 (2017) 693–704
http://dx.doi.org/10.1016/j.hoc.2017.04.004
0889-8588/17/© 2017 Elsevier Inc. All rights reserved.

3 Over the past several decades, a great deal of work has been invested in the development of large arsenals of small molecules that can potently and selectively block the activity of many specific kinases.[7]

Effective translation of this diverse collection of small-molecule kinase inhibitors into a clinical setting requires an understanding of the individual patients and larger patient populations most likely to benefit from different kinase inhibitors. This task is more complex than it might seem, because the routes to kinase pathway dysregulation are numerous and far more complex than a simple genomic lesion in the kinase of interest. Some of these routes are listed as follows, with examples of each taken from the hematologic malignancy literature.

Chromosomal Translocation

Chronic myeloid leukemia (CML) is caused by the 9;22 chromosomal translocation, resulting in the BCR-ABL fusion gene.[8–18] The same BCR-ABL gene fusion has also been implicated in adult and pediatric acute lymphoblastic leukemia (ALL),[19,20] and more recently a wider diversity of tyrosine kinase gene fusions have been reported in ALL cases with similar gene expression signature, but lacking the BCR-ABL–causing chromosomal rearrangement.[21] In addition, there are numerous rearrangements involving fusions of genes in other gene families in hematologic malignancies, and some of these have been reported to lead indirectly to kinase pathway dysregulation.[22–25]

Point Mutations and Insertion/Deletions

One of the best examples of point mutations and insertion/deletions playing a prominent role in hematologic malignancies comes from the myeloproliferative neoplasms, polycythemia vera, primary myelofibrosis, and essential thrombocythemia, in which most cases were found to have point mutations in *JAK2* or *MPL*.[26–34] Subsequently, frameshift mutations in *CALR* were found in most *JAK2/MPL* wild-type cases, and these frame-shifted *CALR* mutants were shown to interact with and dysregulate MPL/JAK2 signaling.[35–38] Importantly, this example shows that genetic lesions affecting any number of genes in nonkinase gene families can still lead to kinase pathway dysregulation through complex mechanisms.

Aberrant Expression

Aberrant expression of kinases has been reported in numerous cancers with one of the best-known examples arising from amplification of ERBB2 (HER2) in breast cancer, and examples also exist in hematologic malignancies, such as upregulation of hepatocyte growth factor and its receptor tyrosine kinase, MET, in acute myeloid leukemia (AML).[39]

Oncorequisite Pathways

Although there are numerous examples of a kinase pathway that becomes dysregulated due to a genetic or epigenetic event, there are also emerging examples of pathways that are critical for tumor cell growth and viability without overt alterations in the sequence or expression level of these genes, and specific examples indicate these pathways can be successfully targeted. One of the best examples of this from hematologic malignancies comes from the lymphoid tumors in which the B-cell receptor, which is not mutated and naturally expressed in lymphomas at levels similar to normal B cells, has been demonstrated to be targetable with inhibitors of BCR-associated kinases such as BTK, SRC-family kinases, or SYK.[40–46] Similar findings have also been made in subsets of ALL cases that similarly depend on the pre-BCR.[24,47]

Microenvironment

Finally, the tumor microenvironment has been demonstrated to provide critical signals maintaining tumor cell growth and viability, and many of these signals proceed through kinase pathways. Prominent examples in the hematologic malignancies include tumor necrosis factor-alpha in myeloproliferative neoplasms,[48] interleukin (IL)-1 in CML,[49,50] and CSF1 in chronic myelomonocytic leukemia.[51]

FUNCTIONAL SCREENING AS A TOOL TO UNDERSTAND KINASE PATHWAY DYSREGULATION

As detailed previously, there are numerous examples of genetic, epigenetic, and microenvironmental routes to kinase pathway dysregulation that have been discovered in hematologic malignancies. However, there is also evidence that kinase pathway dysregulation is operational in a much larger fraction of cases than can be explained by the previously described insights. In 70% to 90% of patients with AML, blast cells exhibit phosphorylation of signal transducer and activator of transcription 5, a marker for tyrosine kinase activity.[52–54] Known kinase pathway alterations can only be explained in approximately 50% of cases at most.[55] Thus, tyrosine kinases have been shown to play a role in the pathogenesis of numerous hematologic malignancies, and there remain a large number of cases that exhibit abnormal tyrosine kinase activity due to mechanisms that have yet to be uncovered. Indeed, recent Phase III clinical trial results testing the multi-kinase inhibitor, midostaurin, in patients with AML with or without mutation of FLT3 showed equivalent benefit for patients with and without FLT3 mutation,[56] suggesting unknown kinase pathways that are targeted by midostaurin are operational in FLT3 wild-type cases.

Hence, although the previously described discoveries have led to clinical exploration of kinase inhibitors on the basis of genetic markers in certain patient subsets, scientific and clinical results have suggested that the application of kinase inhibitors may be more broadly effective than just within these genetically defined subsets. One approach for understanding of kinase pathway dysregulation in cancer is the ex vivo testing of primary patient specimens with panels of small-molecule kinase inhibitors. This approach is appealing for a variety of reasons, including speed of obtaining results (4 days or less) and success of identifying pathway dysregulation irrespective of mechanistic understanding. This latter advantage is particularly important because of the plethora of mechanisms by which kinases have been and could be found to be dysregulated in myeloid malignancies and other cancer subtypes. As detailed later in this article, there are many examples in which kinase inhibitor functional screening has been used to identify novel targets in patients with myeloid malignancy and in some instances, integration of these functional screening data with genomic information has led to new understanding of the mechanistic etiology of kinase pathway dependence.

Kinase Inhibitor Screening to Identify Pathway Dependence in Individual Patients

Functional screening with kinase inhibitors can be useful to identify candidate drugs that can be applied on an individualized basis (**Fig. 1**). One early example of this came in the form of a patient with systemic mastocytosis with associated monocytic leukemia. In this case, screening with panels of small interfering RNAs (siRNAs) and kinase inhibitors revealed dramatic sensitivity of circulating neoplastic monocytes to

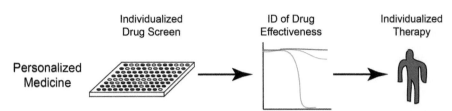

Fig. 1. Functional screening for personalized medicine. Analysis of tumor cells from individual patients can reveal candidate drugs that are effective irrespective of knowledge of the mechanism of drug efficacy. Functional screening results can be obtained within 4 days or less, facilitating clinical translation of data.

silencing or inhibition of JAK2. This led to sequencing of JAK2 and upstream receptors and the identification of a novel insertional mutation in the thrombopoietin receptor, MPL, which was confirmed as a transforming variant of MPL that caused dysregulation of JAK2 signaling. This patient was eligible for a clinical trial with the broad-spectrum kinase inhibitor, midostaurin, which was confirmed to inhibit viability of this patient's cells and to block JAK2 signaling downstream of this transforming variant of MPL. The patient exhibited a dramatic clinical response to midostaurin.[57] Interestingly, this variant of MPL has never been reported in any other patient, confirming the capacity of functional screening to identify actionable kinase pathway targets, even in circumstances of exceedingly rare, unknown genetic lesions.

Cohort-Based Kinase Inhibitor Screening

Functional screening with kinase inhibitors also has been used more broadly to survey larger cohorts of patients, thereby understanding both individual patient specimen responses as well as larger patterns in overall patient cohorts (**Fig. 2**). In 2 of the earliest instances, 2 independent screening platforms applied to 2 distinct patient populations revealed strikingly similar patterns of drug sensitivity, and both studies successfully correlated ex vivo drug response data with clinical responses to targeted therapies.[58,59]

Common Pathways/Drugs for Disease Subsets

In addition to understanding the diversity of responses across cohorts of patient specimens, kinase inhibitor screening has also been used to understand and confirm common patterns of pathway dependence in defined diagnostic hem malignancy subsets (see **Fig. 2**). Examples include the confirmation that the multi-kinase/ABL/SRC/FLT3 inhibitor,

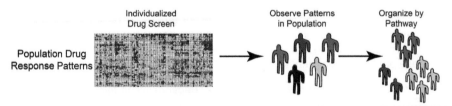

Fig. 2. Functional screening for population and pathway analyses. Screening with kinase inhibitors across larger cohorts of patients can reveal a diversity of patterns of functional drug responses. Organization of these drug responses by pathway of drug targets can reveal dysregulated pathways in distinct patient subsets (eg, B-cell receptor signaling in lymphoid malignancies, JAK pathway signaling in biallelic CEBPA mutant AML).

ponatinib, is indeed effective against patients with AML with FLT3-ITD,[60] and the PI3K-delta inhibitor, idelalisib, is broadly effective in chronic lymphocytic leukemia.[40]

Drug Repurposing

In addition, kinase inhibitor screening has, in some cases, led to surprising discovery that certain drugs can be repurposed for very specific clinical situations. One example of this comes with CML cases with mutation of T315I in the kinase domain of BCR-ABL. Before this study, the only inhibitor approved by the Food and Drug Administration with activity against BCR-ABL T315I was ponatinib; however, kinase inhibitor screening of CML patient samples revealed that cases with T315I were preferentially sensitivity to the kinase inhibitor, axitinib. Subsequent studies revealed that axitinib is preferentially active against the T315I variant of BCR-ABL relative to native BCR-ABL, and these studies have suggested that axitinib, alone or in combination with other ABL kinase inhibitors, may be an effective therapeutic option for patients with T315I-positive CML.[61] Another example of drug repurposing has come from recent studies of AML with biallelic *CEBPA* mutation in which functional sensitivity to JAK kinase inhibitors was correlated with a JAK kinase gene expression signature, as well as mutation of JAK pathway nodes.[62,63]

Kinase Inhibitor Screening to Refine Diagnostic and Therapeutic Markers

In addition to understanding of specific kinase inhibitor sensitivity in individual patients and the diversity of responses across populations, kinase inhibitor screening has also been used identify consistent and heretofore unknown kinase pathway dysregulation within distinct clinical patient subsets (**Fig. 3**). One prominent example comes with the discovery of JAK and SRC-family pathway sensitivity in Philadelphia-negative neutrophilic leukemia cases downstream of somatic mutation of CSF3R (G-CSFR). The 2001 World Health Organization's guidelines for diagnostic subsets of myeloid malignancies restricted classification of CML only to cases exhibiting the 9;22, Philadelphia chromosome rearrangement (Ph).[64] A small number of patients exhibited disease that was clinically similar to CML, but was Ph-negative. For some time, the genetic etiology of these Ph-negative neutrophilic leukemias (chronic neutrophilic leukemia [CNL]; atypical CML [aCML]) remained unknown. Kinase inhibitor screening of patients with CNL revealed sensitivity to JAK and/or SRC-family kinase inhibitors, which corresponded to novel mutations in CSF3R, identified by genomic analyses of these cases.[65] The CSF3R mutations segregated into 2 classes: membrane proximal mutations, which corresponded to JAK inhibitor sensitivity, and cytoplasmic truncating mutations, similar to those observed in a subset of patients with congenital neutropenia,

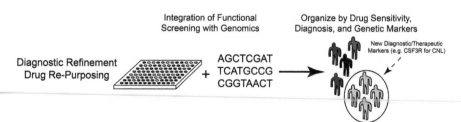

Fig. 3. Functional screening for biomarker discovery and drug repurposing. When combining functional screening with genomic approaches, data integration can help to further organize the evidence of pathway dysregulation around specific genetic biomarkers (eg, CSF3R mutations driving JAK pathway activation in CNL).

which corresponded to sensitivity to SRC-family kinase inhibitors.[66] A syngeneic, bone marrow transplant model of CSF3R mutation recapitulated CNL disease phenotype, which was mitigated with JAK inhibitor treatment.[67] These findings ultimately led to the discovery that CSF3R mutations are highly prevalent in patients with CNL and are observed with lower frequency in patients with aCML. In the recent update to World Health Organization diagnostic guidelines, CSF3R mutation has been included as a diagnostic feature of CNL.[68] Functional screening platforms also can be extensible to other families of small-molecule inhibitors to make similar types of discoveries, such as the recent identification of a HOX gene expression signature as a marker of sensitivity to BH3 mimetics.[69]

Application of Functional Kinase Inhibitor Screening in Lymphoid Malignancies

Although much work has been performed with functional kinase inhibitor screening in myeloid malignancies, there also have been major advances using this approach in the lymphoid setting. Although this review is primarily oriented toward myeloid malignancies, it is useful to also mention the important parallel work ongoing with lymphoid malignancies.

A combination of functional screening with siRNA and kinase inhibitors led to the novel understanding that acute lymphoblastic leukemia cases with a 1;19-chromosomal rearrangement exhibit sensitivity to the cell surface pseudokinase, ROR1, as well as to small molecules that target kinases downstream of the pre–B-cell receptor.[24] More recent work has also shown this disease subset to be sensitive to the PI3K-delta inhibitor, idelalisib, consistent with pre-BCR dependence in this disease subset as well as data showing that the TCF3-PBX1 fusion, which is generated by the 1;19 translocation, upregulates PI3K-delta.[70] This observation was also extended into the highly rare, but extremely aggressive subset of patients with 17;19 rearrangements, with 1 patient being successfully, although transiently, treated with one of these pre–B-cell receptor kinase inhibitors (dasatinib).[71] Subsequent work revealed that the pre–B-cell receptor pathway is activated and important in an even larger subset of pediatric ALL cases, as many as 10% to 15% of total cases.[47] Further functional screening work revealed that 17;19-rearranged cases are also sensitive to the BCL2 small-molecule inhibitor, venetoclax.[72] Functional screening has also been also been used in the setting of ALL to identify subsets of cases with a high degree of sensitivity to emerging agents, such as SMAC mimetics.[73]

In the setting of T-lineage ALL, functional screening work revealed a heretofore unknown pathway dependence on the cytoplasmic JAK-family kinase TYK2, signaling through STAT1 to enhance BCL2 prosurvival signaling. This was due to an autocrine IL-10 signaling loop in these cells.[74]

Drug Combinations

In addition to the exploration of single-agent efficacy in individual patients and diagnostic subsets, functional screening is also more recently being used to understand potential drug interactions and drug synergies. One notable example comes from a recent study evaluating kinase inhibitors in combination with the small-molecule, homoharringtonine. This study identified synergy of FLT3 inhibitors with homoharringtonine in patients with AML with FLT3-ITD. The results of the functional screening data were used as a springboard for a Phase II clinical trial testing this drug combination in patients with FLT3-ITD–positive AML, and the clinical trial demonstrated clinical efficacy of this drug combination, which correlated with ex vivo functional screening data.[75] Much additional work of this type is needed to understand pairwise drug interactions, which will be even more complex to understand from a genetic and mechanistic perspective than single-agent efficacy (**Fig. 4**).

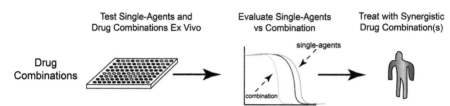

Fig. 4. Functional screening to identify drug combinations. In many disease subsets, successful clinical application of kinase inhibitors will likely require combination with other kinase inhibitors or other drug classes. Functional screening can be a useful tool in identifying the most promising from the myriad of possible drug combinations. By screening single agents and pairwise combinations, chosen from computational predictions, biological insights, or through random selection, ex vivo screening can identify combinations that significantly outperform both single agents. Clinical testing of the efficacy of these synergistic drug combinations is just beginning, but initial trials point to early success (eg, homoharringtonine combined with FLT3 inhibitors for FLT3-mutant AML).

Beyond Kinase Inhibitors

In the previous examples of functional screening, there are already a few instances in which this type of analysis has informed drugs beyond kinase inhibitors. As exciting new drug classes emerge (eg, BH3 and SMAC mimetics, bromodomain inhibitors, metabolic pathway modulators, epigenetic pathway modulators), this form of experimental investigation can surely be a solid source of knowledge to both identify signals of drug efficacy in individual patients and patient populations as well as to better understand the mechanistic etiology of sensitivity to these other classes of drugs. In addition, the prospect and complexity of drug combinations only increases as these new, exciting molecules come to the forefront.

SUMMARY

The impact of next-generation sequencing technologies on cancer research and cancer therapeutics has been dramatic. However, the translation of genomic findings into clinically meaningful strategies has been substantially limited by a biological gap in understanding of the connections between genetic events and drug sensitivity patterns. One modality that can be useful for bridging this divide as well as delivering stand-alone information about drug application and repurposing is ex vivo functional screening. Over the past decade, several groups have used ex vivo screening platforms to make important discoveries regarding kinase pathway dysregulation and clinical targeting in myeloid malignancies as well as other cancer subtypes. In certain instances, integration with genomic data has further accelerated mechanistic understanding and clinical translation. With the advent of many new and exciting drug classes beyond kinase inhibitors, the potential for ex vivo functional screening to inform broader pathway dysregulation and novel drug combinations is immense. Functional screening should assuredly be considered as an important component of the toolkit for precision medicine in myeloid malignancies and beyond.

REFERENCES

1. Druker BJ, Guilhot F, O'Brien SG, et al. Five-year follow-up of patients receiving imatinib for chronic myeloid leukemia. N Engl J Med 2006;355(23):2408–17.

2. Lynch TJ, Bell DW, Sordella R, et al. Activating mutations in the epidermal growth factor receptor underlying responsiveness of non-small-cell lung cancer to gefitinib. N Engl J Med 2004;350(21):2129–39.

3. Paez JG, Janne PA, Lee JC, et al. EGFR mutations in lung cancer: correlation with clinical response to gefitinib therapy. Science 2004;304(5676):1497–500.

4. Smith I, Procter M, Gelber RD, et al. 2-year follow-up of trastuzumab after adjuvant chemotherapy in HER2-positive breast cancer: a randomised controlled trial. Lancet 2007;369(9555):29–36.

5. Krause DS, Van Etten RA. Tyrosine kinases as targets for cancer therapy. N Engl J Med 2005;353(2):172–87.

6. Paul MK, Mukhopadhyay AK. Tyrosine kinase: role and significance in cancer. Int J Med Sci 2004;1(2):101–15.

7. Zhang J, Yang PL, Gray NS. Targeting cancer with small molecule kinase inhibitors. Nature reviews. Cancer 2009;9(1):28–39.

8. Ben-Neriah Y, Daley GQ, Mes-Masson AM, et al. The chronic myelogenous leukemia-specific P210 protein is the product of the BCR/ABL hybrid gene. Science 1986;233(4760):212–4.

9. Collins SJ, Kubonishi I, Miyoshi I, et al. Altered transcription of the C-ABL oncogene in K-562 and other chronic myelogenous leukemia cells. Science 1984; 225(4657):72–4.

10. Daley GQ, Van Etten RA, Baltimore D. Induction of chronic myelogenous leukemia in mice by the P210BCR/ABL gene of the Philadelphia chromosome. Science 1990;247(4944):824–30.

11. Davis RL, Konopka JB, Witte ON. Activation of the C-ABL oncogene by viral transduction or chromosomal translocation generates altered C-ABL proteins with similar in vitro kinase properties. Mol Cell Biol 1985;5(1):204–13.

12. Gale RP, Canaani E. An 8-kilobase ABL RNA transcript in chronic myelogenous leukemia. Proc Natl Acad Sci U S A 1984;81(18):5648–52.

13. Heisterkamp N, Jenster G, ten Hoeve J, et al. Acute leukaemia in BCR/ABL transgenic mice. Nature 1990;344(6263):251–3.

14. Kelliher MA, McLaughlin J, Witte ON, et al. Induction of a chronic myelogenous leukemia-like syndrome in mice with V-ABL and BCR/ABL. Proc Natl Acad Sci U S A 1990;87(17):6649–53.

15. Nowell PC, Hungerford DA. Chromosome studies on normal and leukemic human leukocytes. J Natl Cancer Inst 1960;25:85–109.

16. Rowley JD. Letter: a new consistent chromosomal abnormality in chronic myelogenous leukaemia identified by quinacrine fluorescence and Giemsa staining. Nature 1973;243(5405):290–3.

17. Sherbenou DW, Druker BJ. Applying the discovery of the Philadelphia chromosome. J Clin Invest 2007;117(8):2067–74.

18. Shtivelman E, Lifshitz B, Gale RP, et al. Fused transcript of ABL and BCR genes in chronic myelogenous leukaemia. Nature 1985;315(6020):550–4.

19. Clark SS, McLaughlin J, Crist WM, et al. Unique forms of the ABL tyrosine kinase distinguish Ph1-positive CML from Ph1-positive ALL. Science 1987;235(4784): 85–8.

20. Uckun FM, Nachman JB, Sather HN, et al. Clinical significance of Philadelphia chromosome positive pediatric acute lymphoblastic leukemia in the context of contemporary intensive therapies: a report from the Children's Cancer Group. Cancer 1998;83(9):2030–9.

21. Roberts KG, Li Y, Payne-Turner D, et al. Targetable kinase-activating lesions in Ph-like acute lymphoblastic leukemia. N Engl J Med 2014;371(11):1005–15.

22. Armstrong SA, Kung AL, Mabon ME, et al. Inhibition of FLT3 in MLL. Validation of a therapeutic target identified by gene expression based classification. Cancer Cell 2003;3(2):173–83.

23. Armstrong SA, Staunton JE, Silverman LB, et al. MLL translocations specify a distinct gene expression profile that distinguishes a unique leukemia. Nat Genet 2002;30(1):41–7.

24. Bicocca VT, Chang BH, Masouleh BK, et al. Crosstalk between ROR1 and the pre-B-cell receptor promotes survival of t(1;19) acute lymphoblastic leukemia. Cancer Cell 2012;2012(22):656–67.

25. Yeoh EJ, Ross ME, Shurtleff SA, et al. Classification, subtype discovery, and prediction of outcome in pediatric acute lymphoblastic leukemia by gene expression profiling. Cancer Cell 2002;1(2):133–43.

26. Baxter EJ, Scott LM, Campbell PJ, et al. Acquired mutation of the tyrosine kinase JAK2 in human myeloproliferative disorders. Lancet 2005;365(9464):1054–61.

27. James C, Ugo V, Le Couedic JP, et al. A unique clonal JAK2 mutation leading to constitutive signalling causes polycythaemia vera. Nature 2005;434(7037): 1144–8.

28. Kralovics R, Passamonti F, Buser AS, et al. A gain-of-function mutation of JAK2 in myeloproliferative disorders. N Engl J Med 2005;352(17):1779–90.

29. Levine RL, Wadleigh M, Cools J, et al. Activating mutation in the tyrosine kinase JAK2 in polycythemia vera, essential thrombocythemia, and myeloid metaplasia with myelofibrosis. Cancer Cell 2005;7(4):387–97.

30. Quentmeier H, MacLeod RA, Zaborski M, et al. JAK2 V617F tyrosine kinase mutation in cell lines derived from myeloproliferative disorders. Leukemia 2006; 20(3):471–6.

31. Walters DK, Goss VL, Stoffregen EP, et al. Phosphoproteomic analysis of AML cell lines identifies leukemic oncogenes. Leuk Res 2006;30:1097–104.

32. Wernig G, Mercher T, Okabe R, et al. Expression of Jak2V617F causes a polycythemia vera-like disease with associated myelofibrosis in a murine bone marrow transplant model. Blood 2006;107(11):4274–81.

33. Zhao R, Xing S, Li Z, et al. Identification of an acquired JAK2 mutation in polycythemia vera. J Biol Chem 2005;280(24):22788–92.

34. Pikman Y, Lee BH, Mercher T, et al. MPLW515L is a novel somatic activating mutation in myelofibrosis with myeloid metaplasia. PLoS Med 2006;3(7):e270.

35. Araki M, Yang Y, Masubuchi N, et al. Activation of the thrombopoietin receptor by mutant calreticulin in CALR-mutant myeloproliferative neoplasms. Blood 2016; 127(10):1307–16.

36. Elf S, Abdelfattah NS, Chen E, et al. Mutant calreticulin requires both its mutant C-terminus and the thrombopoietin receptor for oncogenic transformation. Cancer Discov 2016;6(4):368–81.

37. Garbati MR, Welgan CA, Landefeld SH, et al. Mutant calreticulin-expressing cells induce monocyte hyperreactivity through a paracrine mechanism. Am J Hematol 2016;91(2):211–9.

38. Marty C, Pecquet C, Nivarthi H, et al. Calreticulin mutants in mice induce an MPL-dependent thrombocytosis with frequent progression to myelofibrosis. Blood 2016;127(10):1317–24.

39. Kentsis A, Reed C, Rice KL, et al. Autocrine activation of the MET receptor tyrosine kinase in acute myeloid leukemia. Nat Med 2012;18(7):1118–22.

40. Lannutti BJ, Meadows SA, Herman SE, et al. CAL-101, a p110delta selective phosphatidylinositol-3-kinase inhibitor for the treatment of B-cell malignancies, inhibits PI3K signaling and cellular viability. Blood 2011;117(2):591–4.

41. Herman SE, Gordon AL, Wagner AJ, et al. Phosphatidylinositol 3-kinase-delta inhibitor CAL-101 shows promising preclinical activity in chronic lymphocytic leukemia by antagonizing intrinsic and extrinsic cellular survival signals. Blood 2011; 116(12):2078–88.

42. Stevenson FK, Krysov S, Davies AJ, et al. B-cell receptor signaling in chronic lymphocytic leukemia. Blood 2011;118(16):4313–20.

43. Rodriguez A, Villuendas R, Yanez L, et al. Molecular heterogeneity in chronic lymphocytic leukemia is dependent on BCR signaling: clinical correlation. Leukemia 2007;21(9):1984–91.

44. Byrd JC, Furman RR, Coutre SE, et al. Targeting BTK with ibrutinib in relapsed chronic lymphocytic leukemia. N Engl J Med 2013;369(1):32–42.

45. Brown JR, Byrd JC, Coutre SE, et al. Idelalisib, an inhibitor of phosphatidylinositol 3-kinase p110delta, for relapsed/refractory chronic lymphocytic leukemia. Blood 2014;123(22):3390–7.

46. Friedberg JW, Sharman J, Sweetenham J, et al. Inhibition of Syk with fostamatinib disodium has significant clinical activity in non-Hodgkin lymphoma and chronic lymphocytic leukemia. Blood 2010;115(13):2578–85.

47. Geng H, Hurtz C, Lenz KB, et al. Self-enforcing feedback activation between BCL6 and pre-B cell receptor signaling defines a distinct subtype of acute lymphoblastic leukemia. Cancer Cell 2015;27(3):409–25.

48. Fleischman AG, Aichberger KJ, Luty SB, et al. TNFalpha facilitates clonal expansion of JAK2V617F positive cells in myeloproliferative neoplasms. Blood 2011; 118(24):6392–8.

49. Bhatia R, McGlave PB, Dewald GW, et al. Abnormal function of the bone marrow microenvironment in chronic myelogenous leukemia: role of malignant stromal macrophages. Blood 1995;85(12):3636–45.

50. Zhang B, Chu S, Agarwal P, et al. Inhibition of interleukin-1 signaling enhances elimination of tyrosine kinase inhibitor treated CML stem cells. Blood 2016; 128(23):2671–82.

51. Obba S, Hizir Z, Boyer L, et al. The PRKAA1/AMPKalpha1 pathway triggers autophagy during CSF1-induced human monocyte differentiation and is a potential target in CMML. Autophagy 2015;11(7):1114–29.

52. Birkenkamp KU, Geugien M, Lemmink HH, et al. Regulation of constitutive STAT5 phosphorylation in acute myeloid leukemia blasts. Leukemia 2001;15(12): 1923–31.

53. Hayakawa F, Towatari M, Iida H, et al. Differential constitutive activation between STAT-related proteins and MAP kinase in primary acute myelogenous leukaemia. Br J Haematol 1998;101(3):521–8.

54. Spiekermann K, Pau M, Schwab R, et al. Constitutive activation of STAT3 and STAT5 is induced by leukemic fusion proteins with protein tyrosine kinase activity and is sufficient for transformation of hematopoietic precursor cells. Exp Hematol 2002;30(3):262–71.

55. Cancer Genome Atlas Research Network, Ley TJ, Miller C, Ding L, et al. Genomic and epigenomic landscapes of adult de novo acute myeloid leukemia. N Engl J Med 2013;368(22):2059–74.

56. Stone RM, Mandrekar S, Sanford BL, et al. The multi-kinase inhibitor midostaurin (M) prolongs survival compared with placebo (P) in combination with daunorubicin (D)/cytarabine (C) induction (ind), high-dose C consolidation (consol), and as maintenance (maint) therapy in newly diagnosed acute myeloid leukemia (AML) patients (pts) age 18–60 with FLT3 mutations (muts): an international

prospective randomized (rand) P-controlled double-blind trial (CALGB 10603/ RATIFY [Alliance]). Blood 2015;126(23):6. ASH Supplement.

57. Tyner JW, Deininger MW, Loriaux MM, et al. RNAi screen for rapid therapeutic target identification in leukemia patients. Proc Natl Acad Sci U S A 2009; 106(21):8695–700.

58. Pemovska T, Kontro M, Yadav B, et al. Individualized systems medicine strategy to tailor treatments for patients with chemorefractory acute myeloid leukemia. Cancer Discov 2013;3(12):1416–29.

59. Tyner JW, Yang WF, Bankhead A, et al. Kinase pathway dependence in primary human leukemias determined by rapid inhibitor screening. Cancer Res 2013; 73(1):285–96.

60. Gozgit JM, Wong MJ, Wardwell S, et al. Potent activity of ponatinib (AP24534) in models of FLT3-driven acute myeloid leukemia and other hematologic malignancies. Mol Cancer Ther 2011;10(6):1028–35.

61. Pemovska T, Johnson E, Kontro M, et al. Axitinib effectively inhibits BCR-ABL1(T315I) with a distinct binding conformation. Nature 2015;519(7541): 102–5.

62. Lavallee VP, Krosl J, Lemieux S, et al. Chemo-genomic interrogation of CEBPA mutated AML reveals recurrent CSF3R mutations and subgroup sensitivity to JAK inhibitors. Blood 2016;127(24):3054–61.

63. Maxson JE, Ries RE, Wang YC, et al. CSF3R mutations have a high degree of overlap with CEBPA mutations in pediatric AML. Blood 2016;127(24):3094–8.

64. Jaffe ES, Harris NL, Stein H, et al, editors. World Health Organization classification of tumours: pathology and genetics of tumours of haematopoietic and lymphoid tissues. Lyon (France): IARC; 2001.

65. Maxson JE, Gotlib J, Pollyea DA, et al. Oncogenic CSF3R mutations in chronic neutrophilic leukemia and atypical CML. N Engl J Med 2013;368(19):1781–90.

66. Maxson JE, Luty SB, Macmaniman J, et al. Ligand-independence of the colony stimulating factor 3 receptor (CSF3R) T618I mutation results from loss of O-linked glycosylation and increased receptor dimerization. J Biol Chem 2014;289(9): 5820–7.

67. Fleischman AG, Maxson JE, Luty SB, et al. The CSF3R T618I mutation causes a lethal neutrophilic neoplasia in mice that is responsive to therapeutic JAK inhibition. Blood 2013;122(22):3628–31.

68. Arber DA, Orazi A, Hasserjian R, et al. The 2016 revision to the World Health Organization classification of myeloid neoplasms and acute leukemia. Blood 2016;127(20):2391–405.

69. Kontro M, Kumar A, Majumder MM, et al. HOX gene expression predicts response to BCL-2 inhibition in acute myeloid leukemia. Leukemia 2017;31(2): 301–9.

70. Eldfors S, Kuusanmaki H, Kontro M, et al. Idelalisib sensitivity and mechanisms of disease progression in relapsed TCF3-PBX1 acute lymphoblastic leukemia. Leukemia 2017;31(1):51–7.

71. Glover JM, Loriaux M, Tyner JW, et al. In vitro sensitivity to dasatinib in lymphoblasts from a patient with t(17;19)(q22;p13) gene rearrangement pre-B acute lymphoblastic leukemia. Pediatr Blood Cancer 2011;59(3):576–9.

72. Fischer U, Forster M, Rinaldi A, et al. Genomics and drug profiling of fatal TCF3-HLF-positive acute lymphoblastic leukemia identifies recurrent mutation patterns and therapeutic options. Nat Genet 2015;47(9):1020–9.

73. McComb S, Aguade-Gorgorio J, Harder L, et al. Activation of concurrent apoptosis and necroptosis by SMAC mimetics for the treatment of refractory and relapsed ALL. Sci Transl Med 2016;8(339):339ra70.

74. Sanda T, Tyner JW, Gutierrez A, et al. TYK2-STAT1-BCL2 pathway dependence in T-cell acute lymphoblastic leukemia. Cancer Discov 2013;3(5):564–77.

75. Lam SS, Ho ES, He BL, et al. Homoharringtonine (omacetaxine mepesuccinate) as an adjunct for FLT3-ITD acute myeloid leukemia. Sci Transl Med 2016;8(359): 359ra129.

Identification and Targeting of Kinase Alterations in Histiocytic Neoplasms

Neval Ozkaya, MD[a], Ahmet Dogan, MD, PhD[a],
Omar Abdel-Wahab, MD[b],*

KEYWORDS

- ARAF • BRAF • Erdheim-Chester disease • Langerhans cell histiocytosis
- MAP kinase • MEK

KEY POINTS

- Nearly every patient with Langerhans cell histiocytosis and Erdheim-Chester disease has ERK activation owing to activating mutations in ARAF, BRAF, MEK1/2, or N/KRAS, or kinase fusions.
- BRAF inhibition results in dramatic and durable responses in patients with *BRAF* V600E mutant histiocytosis.
- MEK inhibitors may be efficacious for treating *BRAF*-wild-type histiocytosis.
- The safety and therapeutic usefulness of targeted therapy versus conventional therapy for children with Langerhans cell histiocytosis remains to be determined.
- Further genomic analyses are needed to define fusions in patients without point mutations in kinases and those alterations that cooperate with kinase mutations in histiocytoses.

INTRODUCTION

The histiocytoses are a diverse group of disorders defined by the pathologic infiltration of normal tissues by cells of the mononuclear phagocyte system. Owing to biologic variability of the cells of the mononuclear phagocyte system and the tissues they inhabit, histiocytic disorders are among the most intriguing yet complex areas of modern hematology and can be tremendously difficult to diagnose. Until recently, the mechanisms of pathogenesis of the histiocytoses have been speculative and debate

Disclosure Statement: Nothing to disclose.
[a] Department of Pathology, Memorial Sloan Kettering Cancer Center, 1275 York Avenue, New York, NY 10065, USA; [b] Human Oncology and Pathogenesis Program, Memorial Sloan Kettering Cancer Center, 1275 York Avenue, New York, NY 10065, USA
* Corresponding author.
E-mail address: abdelwao@mskcc.org

has focused on the classification of these conditions as reactive versus neoplastic. However, starting 6 years ago, a series of recurrent, activating mutations in genes encoding kinases of the mitogen-activated protein (MAP) kinase (MAPK) system have been discovered in a large proportion of histiocytosis patients. These discoveries have resulted in potently effective therapies in genetically defined subsets of adults with these disorders. Here, we review the recent molecular advances in the systemic histiocytoses and their impact on treatment.

SYSTEMIC HISTIOCYTIC NEOPLASMS AND THEIR CURRENT CLASSIFICATION

According to the fourth edition of the World Health Organization (WHO) classification, histiocytic disorders can be classified into 2 main categories based on the phenotype of cells present within the lesions: (1) Langerhans cell histiocytosis (LCH) and (2) non-Langerhans cell histiocytoses (non-LCH) (**Fig. 1**A). LCH received its name as the tumoral cells share unique ultrastructural features of normal Langerhans cells (LCs). However, comparisons of gene expression between LCH cells and LCs indicate that LCH cells are considerable less mature than LCs and are phenotypically closer to myeloid dendritic cells than they are to LCs.[1,2] These data question LCs as the cell-of-origin of LCH, a hypothesis that has largely been discarded in recent years in favor of the idea that LCH arises from either myeloid dendritic cells, their progenitors, or cells even before dendritic cell, monocyte, or macrophage differentiation.[3]

In the WHO classification system, Langerhans cell lesions are divided into 2 subgroups based on the degree of cytologic atypia and clinical aggressiveness: LCH and Langerhans cell sarcoma. In contrast, non-LCH are a heterogenous group of disorders including Erdheim-Chester disease (ECD), juvenile xanthogranulomatous disease (JXG), Rosai-Dorfman disease (RDD), histiocytic sarcoma (HS), indeterminate cell histiocytosis, and others defined by the accumulation of histiocytes that do not meet the diagnostic criteria for LCH, Langerhans cell sarcoma, or hemophagocytic lymphohistiocytosis (see **Fig. 1**A).[4]

In addition to the WHO Classification, the Histiocyte Society has recently proposed a new classification of histiocytosis incorporating clinicopathologic, prognostic, and new genetic findings that have not been accounted for in the WHO classification. This new classification system categorizes the histiocytoses into 5 groups: "L" (Langerhans), "C" (cutaneous and mucocutaneous), "M" (malignant), "R" (Rosai-Dorfman), and "H" (hemophagocytic) groups[5] (see **Fig. 1**B). One important motivation of this effort to regroup the histiocytoses was to take into considerable new molecular genetic information that has revealed the unexpected genetic similarity between LCH and the non-LCH neoplasms (see **Fig. 1**C, D). Thus, in the revised Histiocyte Society classification, the L group includes LCH and ECD, entities that share mutations in the MAPK pathway in greater than 80% of cases[6,7] and may coexist.[8] This review focuses on the biological and therapeutic importance of MAPK mutations in diseases within this L category. The pathophysiology of hemophagocytic disorders of the H group seem to be distinct from those of the L group disorders and the conditions within the C, M, and R groups do not have clearly defined molecular characteristics of pathophysiology currently.

DISCOVERY OF *B-RAF* PROTOONCOGENE MUTATIONS IN HISTIOCYTOSES

In 2010, Badalian-Very and colleagues[6] identified that 57% of LCH patients carry the *BRAF* V600E mutation, thereby identifying a clonal marker of the disease and suggesting that LCH is driven by activation of the MAPK pathway. This high frequency of *BRAF* V600E mutations was then validated in a subsequent study in LCH[7] and also found in a

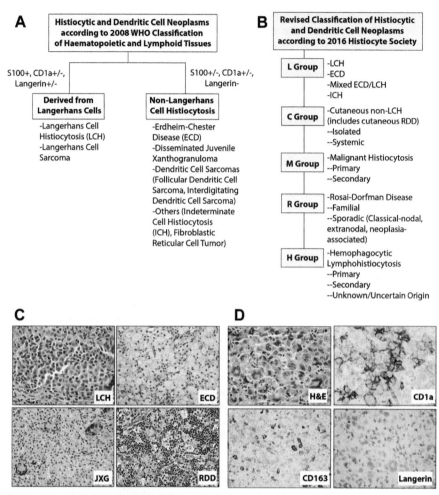

Fig. 1. Characteristic histology of histiocytic lesions. Classification schema for the histiocytoses based on (*A*) the 2008 World Health Organization (WHO) classification and (*B*) a recently updated 2016 classification system from the Histiocyte Society. (*C*) Diagnostic biopsy specimens of Langerhans cell histiocytosis (LCH), Erdheim-Chester disease (ECD), juvenile xanthogranulomatous disease (JXG), and Rosai-Dorfman disease (RDD) lesions stained with hematoxylin and eosin (H&E). The JXG biopsy demonstrates characteristic xanthomatous histiocytes along with multinucleated Touton giant cells. The ECD biopsy shows characteristic infiltration of foamy histiocytes. The LCH biopsy demonstrates characteristic clusters of histiocytes with reniform nuclei and the background inflammatory infiltrate is rich from eosinophils. The RDD biopsy demonstrates characteristic large histiocytes with emperipolesis. (*D*) Diagnostic biopsy specimen for indeterminate cell histiocytosis. H&E stain showing diffuse infiltration by a histiocytic-appearing neoplasm that is indistinguishable from a histiocytic sarcoma by conventional histopathology. Multinucleated cells are seen. The lesion is positive for CD1a and negative for CD163 (reactive histiocytes show positive staining) and Langerin. By definition, neoplastic cells lack Birbeck granules on ultrastructural examination (not shown). (*Data from* [*A*] Swerdlow SH, Campo E, Harris NL, et al. WHO classification of tumours of haematopoietic and lymphoid tissues, vol. 2. 4th edition. WHO Press; 2008; and [*B*] Emile JF, Abla O, Fraitag S, et al. Revised classification of histiocytoses and neoplasms of the macrophage-dendritic cell lineages. Blood 2016;127(22):2672–81.)

significant proportion of patients with non-LCH disorders including approximately 50% of patients with ECD[7] as well as patients with HS.[9] In contrast with recurrent *BRAF* V600E mutations, activating point mutations in *BRAF* other than V600E have been found only rarely in histiocytoses. These include *BRAF* V600D in LCH,[10,11] *BRAFF595L* in HS,[12] and *BRAF V600insDLAT* in LCH.[13] In a recently published study, whole exome sequencing and targeted BRAF sequencing studies in 24 LCH patient samples lacking *BRAF* V600E mutations identified in-frame *BRAF* deletions in the β3-αC loop of BRAF in approximately 6% of LCH patients.[14] This finding identifies *BRAF* deletions as the third most common MAPK pathway alteration in LCH. Importantly, unlike *BRAF* V600E mutant cells, cells bearing *BRAF* in-frame deletions were resistant to the BRAF inhibitor vemurafenib,[14] suggesting a unique biochemical mechanism of ERK activation mediated by different mutations in BRAF. Similar ERK-activating, in-frame *BRAF* deletions have also recently been described in other malignancies including melanoma and ovarian cancers.[15–17]

DISCOVERY OF ADDITIONAL KINASE ALTERATIONS IN HISTIOCYTOSES
A-RAF Protooncogene

After the discovery of *BRAF* V600E mutations in LCH, the consistent identification of phospho-ERK positivity in neoplastic histiocytes in LCH and non-LCH patients regardless of *BRAF* V600E mutational status resulted in an effort to identify additional mutations activating ERK in these orders.[6,18,19] A surprising outcome of 1 whole exome analysis was the discovery of an activating mutation in *ARAF,* an additional RAF kinase, in LCH.[20] *ARAF* mutations have subsequently also been found to be recurrent in non-LCH and are present in 21% of ECD and 12.5% of RDD patients.[21] Although *BRAF* V600E mutations have not been identified in JXG, 18% of JXG cases have been found to have an *ARAF* mutation. However, these activating *ARAF* mutations were found to cooccur with activating *NRAS* mutations in those cases,[21] suggesting that either *ARAF* mutations may occur subclonally in histiocytosis or that they may require additional cooperating activating mutations to drive histiocytosis.

Mitogen-Activated Protein Kinase Kinase 1

Continued genomic analyses of LCH and non-LCH have identified activating mutations in MAPK kinase 1 (*MAP2K1*) as among the most common mutations in the *BRAF* V600-wild-type LCH and non-LCH patients. *MAP2K1* encodes MEK1, the kinase just downstream of the RAF kinases. *MAP2K1* mutations are found only in patients wild type for *BRAF* V600E, consistent with their convergent effects on activation of the MAPK pathway.[19,21,22] The true prevalence of *MAP2K1* mutations in LCH and ECD is uncertain at present because their frequency differs substantially among the samples tested in various reports, which are in between 10% and 40%.[19,21,22] Recently, a *MAP2K1F53L* mutation was identified in an HS lesion, which was possibly transdifferentiated from a follicular lymphoma (as supported by the fact that both lesions harbored a *BCL2* gene rearrangement). In this case, the *MAP2K1* mutation was specific to the HS and not present in the follicular lymphoma, suggesting that the *MAP2K1* mutation may specifically drive the histiocytosis phenotype.[23]

Ras Isoforms

As with other hematologic malignancies, recurrent mutations in *N/KRAS* but not in *HRAS* have been found in systemic histiocytoses. This includes *NRAS* mutations in 3% to 7% of ECD and *NRAS* and *KRAS* mutations in 18% of JXG patients, respectively.[21,24] However, *RAS* mutations frequently coexist with activating *ARAF* mutations in JXG, as discussed. Similarly, *NRAS* and *KRAS* mutations are present in 12.5% and 25% of RDD patients, respectively.[21] The sole exception to the lack of *HRAS* mutations in histiocytosis has been the report of an *HRAS* mutation in an HS with a concomitant *BRAF*F595L mutation.[12] In contrast with non-LCH patients, rare *RAS* mutations have been reported in LCH patients in the setting of concomitant juvenile myelomonocytic leukemia[25] and have not been reported in patients with LCH alone. Although this is a genomic abnormality characteristic of JMML, upregulation of ERK signaling through *NRAS* activation also seems to drive LCH based on human genetic data as well as mouse model phenotypes where the *NRAS*G12D mutation is expressed in hematopoietic cells.[26]

Phosphoinositide 3-Kinases Isoforms

Consistent with potential activation of the PI3K-AKT signaling pathway downstream of *RAS* mutations in non-LCH, *PIK3CA* mutations have been described in 17% of *BRAF*–wild-type ECD patients.[21] These mutations cluster in the α-helical and kinase domains of *PIK3CA*,[21,24] as has been reported in other forms of cancer. Similar to the rarity of *RAS* mutations in LCH, activating mutations in *PIK3CA* have only been identified in 1.2% of LCH patients.[11,27] In addition to *PIK3CA* mutations, rare *PI3KD* mutations have been identified in JXG.[19] In contrast with the consistent role of ERK activation in the histiocytoses, the expression of PI3K isoforms and the role of constitutive PI3K-AKT signaling need to be further evaluated in the pathogenesis of the histiocytoses.

Mitogen-Activated Protein Kinase Kinase Kinase 1

In the course of performing whole exome sequencing on LCH lesions, Nelson and colleagues[22] also discovered 2 somatic mutations in MAPK kinase kinase (*MAP3K1*), which encodes MEKKK1, an enzyme with both E3 ubiquitin ligase activity as well as serine/threonine kinase activity. Both mutations identified in *MAP3K1* in LCH are frameshift deletions leading to truncated proteins (*MAP3K1*T799fs and L1481fs). However, the effects of these mutations on ERK activation are still unclear.

GENE FUSIONS

In addition to single nucleotide variants and small insertion/deletion mutations, structural alterations and gene fusions represent important somatic alterations driving the pathogenesis of common cancers. However, no gene fusions had been uncovered in histiocytic neoplasms until 2015, when 2 studies described gene fusions in *BRAF* V600E-wild-type, non-LCH neoplasms.[21,28] These include an *RNF11-BRAF* fusion in JXG and a *CLIP2-BRAF* fusion in a patient with a non-LCH resembling HS. In both cases, exons 11 to 18 of *BRAF* were involved in the fusion, leading to loss of the N-terminal regulatory, RAS-binding domain of *BRAF* with placement of the intact *BRAF* kinase domain under the aberrant regulation of another promoter. It is not clear what role, if any, the N-terminal fusion partner to *BRAF* may play in these cases. In a recently published paper, Chakraborty and colleagues[14] identified another *BRAF* fusion event involving *FAM73A* (*MIGA1*) on chromosome 1p31.1 and *BRAF* (located on chromosome 7q34) in LCH. The chimeric *FAM73A-BRAF* gene was predicted to result in an in-frame protein lacking the autoinhibitory domain of *BRAF* (exons 1–8) but retaining an intact kinase domain, as has been observed for other known *BRAF* fusion genes.

In addition to *BRAF* fusions, fusions involving *ALK* have been described in 2 ECD patients, both kinesin family member 5B (*KIF5B*)-*ALK* fusions. In both cases, the N-terminal coiled-coil domain of KIF5B was fused to the intact kinase domain of ALK, resulting in inappropriate expression and constitutive activation of ALK.[21]

KIF5B serves as a microtubule-dependent motor involved in the normal distribution of mitochondria and lysosomes, whereas *ALK* encodes a neuronal orphan receptor tyrosine kinase whose expression is normally limited to the nervous system. *KIF5B-ALK* fusions, therefore, result in inappropriate ALK expression and constitutive activation of the MAPK and PI3K-AKT pathways within histiocytes. Similarly, an *EML4-ALK* rearrangement was also more recently described in the lesional biopsy of an adolescent patient with histiocytosis not otherwise specified.[29] Both the *KIF5B-ALK* and *EML4-ALK* fusions have similar configurations to those previously described in non–small-cell lung cancer[30,31] and are functionally activating kinase fusions that show sensitivity to ALK inhibition in vitro.

Thus far, fusions of neurotrophic tyrosine kinase member (neurotrophic tyrosine kinase, receptor type 1 [NTRK1]) have been described in 2 cases of histiocytic neoplasms. In the first case, the lesional biopsy from an ECD patient was confirmed to lead to fusion of the N-terminal coiled-coil domain of Lamin A/C (LMNA) to the intact kinase domain of NTRK1 resulting in inappropriate expression and constitutive activation of NTRK1.[21] *LMNA* encodes a component of the nuclear lamina, a fibrous layer on the inner nuclear membrane that provides a framework for the nuclear envelope. *NTRK1* encodes the TrkA receptor tyrosine kinase, which is a membrane-bound receptor that phosphorylates itself and members of the MAPK pathway leading to cellular proliferation and differentiation. More recently, a *TPR-NTRK1* fusion was detected in an adult patient with histiocytosis not otherwise specified. Both kinase fusions including *LMNA-NTRK1* and *TPR-NTRK1* result in inappropriate expression of NTRK1 with consequent constitutive activation of MAPK and PI3K-AKT pathways within histiocytes. These fusions have similar configurations to previously described *LMNA-NTRK1* fusions in spitzoid neoplasms[32] and *TPR-NTRK1* fusions in lipofibromatosis-like neural tumors.[33] Whether these fusions in ALK or NTRK1 in histiocytosis results in clinical sensitivity to ALK and NTRK inhibitors, respectively, will be important to determine in the near future.

In addition to activating kinase fusions, recurrent Ets variant 3-nuclear receptor coactivator 2 fusions (*ETV3-NCOA2*) fusions have now been described in indeterminate cell histiocytosis.[28] This fusion juxtaposes the N-terminal ETS domain of ETV3, a winged helix-turn-helix DNA-binding domain,[28,34,35] to the C-terminal transcriptional activation domains transcriptional activation domain 1 (AD1), CBP/p300 interaction domain (CID), and transcriptional activation domain 2 (AD2) of NCOA2. This configuration is consistent with previously described *NCOA2* fusions in cancer.[28,34,36–39] Previous studies of *NCOA2* fusions have demonstrated that the AD1 and CID domains are required for the transformation of *NCOA2* fusion proteins.[34,37,39] The involvement of the same NCOA2 C-terminal domains and the evidence that the AD1 and CID domains are necessary for NCOA2 fusion protein transformation supports a model where the NCOA2 C-terminal transcriptional activation domains are targeted aberrantly by the DNA-binding domain provided by an N-terminal fusion partner.[28,34,36–39] It is not yet clear how the *ETV3-NCOA2* fusion relates to the persistent MAPK activation known to be present in indeterminate cell histiocytosis patients. Further functional characterization of the *ETV3-NCOA2* fusion in the pathogenesis of histiocytic neoplasms is, therefore, needed.

THERAPEUTIC EFFICACY OF KINASE INHIBITOR THERAPY IN HISTIOCYTOSES

These molecular advances have led to the advent of clinical studies and trials of targeted molecular therapeutics for patients with histiocytosis described elsewhere in this article (**Fig. 2, Table 1**).

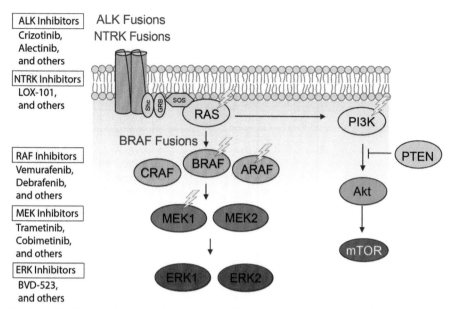

Fig. 2. Activating mutations driving kinase signaling in histiocytic neoplasms. Approximately 50% of patients with Langerhans cell histiocytosis (LCH) and non-LCH neoplasms have a *BRAF*V600E mutation. This is closely followed by mutations in *MAP2K1* (encoding MEK1). Non-LCH patients also have a high frequency of *ARAF* and *N/KRAS* mutations, which are present at lower frequencies in LCH patients. Mutations in *BRAF* outside of V600 residue as well as fusions of *BRAF, ALK,* and *NTRK1* are also known to occur in LCH and non-LCH. Finally, rare activating mutations in PIK3CA are known to occur in LCH and non-LCH. Thus far, there are clinical data supporting the use of RAF inhibitors for *BRAF*V600E mutant histiocytosis and preliminary data to support the use of MEK inhibitors in the use of *BRAF*V600 wild-type histiocytosis. There are no published data regarding the use of ALK, NTRK, or ERK inhibitors in patients with histiocytic disorders. mTOR, mammalian target of rapamycin.

RAF Inhibitors

Clinical experience with the use of BRAF inhibitors for *BRAF* V600E mutant solid tumors motivated use of these same agents for patients with histiocytosis shortly after their discovery. Thus far, the only prospective clinical trial of RAF inhibitors in histiocytosis occurred as part of a histology-independent "basket" study using the BRAF inhibitor vemurafenib for patients with *BRAF* V600E mutant cancers of several different histologic types. In this study, a combined cohort of 22 ECD and 4 LCH patients experienced a response rate of 64% to vemurafenib.[40] Moreover, extended follow-up of this study presented at the 2016 American Society of Hematology meeting has identified that these responses are durable with a median treatment duration now of 14.9 months (range, 2–43).[41] In addition to this clinical trial, a prospective case series by Haroche and colleagues[42] has reported favorable responses to vemurafenib in 8 adult patients with severe, treatment-refractory, *BRAF V600E*-mutant ECD or ECD/LCH mixed histiocytosis. All patients in this study had a significant and sustained clinical response as measured by PET scanning at a median of 10 months (range, 10–16).

In contrast with the results of vemurafenib treatment in adults with histiocytosis, there is only a single report of a child with histiocytosis treated with vemurafenib. In this case, an 8 month old with *BRAF*-mutated, high-risk LCH, whose disease failed

Table 1
Clinical studies and trials of targeted agents for the treatment of histiocytic neoplasms

Clinical Studies and Trials	Therapeutic Agent	Mechanism of Action	Patient Population	Notes
Haroche et al,[42] 2015	Vemurafenib	RAF inhibitor	Eight adult patients with severe, treatment refractory *BRAF*-mutant ECD or ECD/LCH hybrid disease.	All patients had a significant and sustained clinical response as measured by PET scanning during a 6–16-mo follow-up period (mean, 10.5).
Hyman et al,[40] 2015	Vemurafenib	RAF inhibitor	Phase II clinical trial with 18 adults with *BRAF*-mutant ECD or LCH.	43% response rate with 86% of patients showing disease regression. No progression while on treatment (0.6–18.6 mo; median, 5.9).
Gianfreda et al,[50] 2015	Sirolimus	mTOR inhibitor	Open-label trial of 10 patients with ECD	Eight of 10 patients had objective responses or disease stabilization, whereas 2/10 patients had disease progression.
Diamond et al,[21] 2016	Trametinib and cobimetinib	MEK inhibitors	Two adult ECD patients	Dramatic radiologic improvements, as well as clinical improvements. Both patients have been sustained for nearly 6 mo.
Aubart et al,[45] 2016	Cobimetinib	MEK inhibitor	Three *BRAF*-wild-type ECD patients refractory to conventional therapy	All patients had a sustained metabolic response (follow-up of 5–22 mo).

Lee et al,[29] 2017	Trametinib	MEK inhibitor	One adult LCH patient with a *BRAF* inframe-deletion (BRAFN486_P490del).	Dramatic response within 5 d of initiating treatment. Follow-up PET-CT scanning showed complete resolution of lesions.
NCT01677741	Dabrafenib	RAF inhibitor	Ongoing phase I/II trial in children with LCH	One child with refractory LCH treated with oral dabrafenib continued to show stable disease at week 16.
NCT02124772	Trametinib in combination with dabrafenib	RAF and MEK inhibitors	Children and adolescents with *BRAFV600E*-mutant diseases including LCH	
NCT02649972	Cobimetinib	MEK inhibitor	Open-label, single-center, phase II trial for adults with ECD, RDD, ECD/RDD hybrid, LCH with *BRAF*-wild-type histiocytosis or *BRAFV600E*-mutated histiocytosis intolerant of or without access to BRAF inhibitor therapy.	Preliminary results demonstrated robust efficacy.[48] Twenty percent of patients showed a complete metabolic response and 80% a partial metabolic response.
NCT02281760	Dabrafenib and trametinib	RAF and MEK inhibitors	Phase II, open-label trial of dabrafenib and trametinib in adult ECD patients with *BRAFV600E*-mutant lesion.	

Abbreviations: CT, computed tomography; ECD, Erdheim-Chester disease; LCH, Langerhans cell histiocytosis; RDD, Rosai-Dorfman disease.

to respond to multiple rounds of prior therapy, experienced dramatic clinical efficacy to vemurafenib with a sustained response during the 10-month follow-up period.[27] Pediatric formulations are being developed, and phase I/II trials are ongoing in pediatrics with LCH for the first-generation *BRAF* inhibitor, dabrafenib (NCT01677741). Preliminary results describe 2 children with refractory LCH treated with dabrafenib, one of whom had stable disease at week 16.[43]

Although the development of acquired resistance as well as de novo resistance to vemurafenib is commonly observed in *BRAF* V600E-mutant melanoma and other cancers, to date RAF inhibitor resistance has been described in only a single patient with *BRAF* V600E-mutant histiocytosis.[44] In this case, a patient with *BRAF* V600E-mutant ECD without evidence of *MAP2K1* or *N/KRAS* mutations at diagnosis developed acquired dabrafenib resistance coincident with identification of a *KRAS*Q61H-mutant/ *BRAF* V600E-wild-type ECD lesion at clinical relapse. These lesions further regressed with the addition of the MEK inhibitor trametinib to dabrafenib.[44] Notably, a phase II therapeutic trial of the use of dabrafenib, a BRAF V600E inhibitor, and trametinib, an inhibitor of MEK, in ECD patients with BRAF V600E mutation-positive lesions is ongoing (NCT02281760).

MEK Inhibitors

The efficacy of MEK inhibitors for histiocytosis was first reported in 2 non-LCH patients with *MAP2K1*K57N and *MAP2K1*Q56P mutations treated with trametinib and cobimetinib, respectively.[21] Both patients experienced dramatic radiologic improvements, as well as clinical improvements, and both have been sustained for nearly 6 months. Cohen Aubart and colleagues[45] also reported their retrospective results of cobimetinib used in monotherapy for 3 *BRAF*–wild-type patients with ECD. The 3 patients had a sustained metabolic response, and response was assessed with PET scan and also confirmed by decrease of creatinine and C-reactive protein levels and/or MRI. Although 2 of the 3 patients in this study had a *MAP2K1* mutation, the exact mutation was not noted. This is important, because some mutations in *MAP2K1* mutations have been reported as resistant MEK inhibition.[46] Recently, Azorsa and colleagues[47] reported a patient with treatment refractory LCH and identified a novel mutation in the *MAP2K1* gene (*MAP2K1* c.293_310del mutation), which leads to p-ERK activation. This mutation was found to be nonresponsive to a MEK inhibitor in vitro as well as in vivo, because the patient progressed under trametinib treatment.[47] These findings emphasize the importance of functional assessment of genomic data in assigning treatment for patients. In another recent study, an adult LCH patient with PET with fludeoxyglucose F 18 lesions in the neck and groin declined systemic chemotherapy owing to concerns regarding its impact on her quality of life.[29] Targeted sequencing of a biopsy from the neck lesion revealed a *BRAF* inframe deletion (N486_P490del) with a variant allele frequency of 14%. Experimental evidence indicated that akin to *BRAF* V600E, this mutation also results in constitutive activation of downstream signaling but insensitive to V600E-specific inhibitors. Thus, trametinib was started and within 5 days of initiating treatment, her neck and groin tumors disappeared. Follow-up PET-computed tomography showed her lesions had completely resolved.[29]

To determine the therapeutic efficacy of single-agent MEK inhibition in histiocytosis in a prospective fashion, a phase II trial of single-agent cobimetinib for adults with histiocytic disorders is currently ongoing (NCT02649972). This is an open-label, single-center study exploring the efficacy and safety of single-agent cobimetinib in patients with histiocytic disorders whose tumors are *BRAF* V600 wild-type or *BRAF* V600E mutant and are intolerant to, or unable to access, BRAF inhibitors. Preliminary results demonstrated robust efficacy of single-agent cobimetinib in 7 of 7 patients with

BRAF–wild-type ECD, RDD, and LCH on this trial with 20% of patients showing a complete metabolic response and 80% a partial metabolic response. Metabolic response was evaluated by PET with fludeoxyglucose F 18 scan performed every 2 cycles[48] as is commonly performed to radiographically evaluate lesions in histiocytosis patients.

The MEK inhibitor cobimetinib has been evaluated in association with vemurafenib in metastatic melanoma and treatment with both a RAF inhibitor and an MEK1 inhibitor, such as trametinib, may prevent the appearance of resistance.[49] Such a trial of trametinib in combination with dabrafenib in children and adolescents with *BRAF* V600E mutation-positive diseases including LCH has been started (NCT02124772).

Mammalian Target of Rapamycin Inhibitors

In addition to targeting the MAPK pathway, the inflammatory–neoplastic nature of ECD and previously described *PIK3CA* mutations leading to mammalian target of rapamycin pathway activation in 11% of ECD patients[24] has led to efforts to inhibit PI3K signaling in histiocytosis. To this end, a 10-patient trial of the mammalian target of rapamycin inhibitor sirolimus and prednisone was recently reported.[50] Eight patients achieved stable disease or objective responses, whereas 2 had disease progression. Treatment was continued at least 24 months in patients who showed disease stabilization or improvement. Although responses were far less dramatic than those observed in *BRAF*-mutated ECD patients receiving vemurafenib, the therapeutic efficacy of sirolimus and steroids in this trial was not negligible. Moreover, none of the patients in this series harbored *PIK3CA* gain-of-function mutations, suggesting the need to focus PI3K inhibition on the subset of ECD patients that actually carry activating mutations in this pathway.[50]

SUMMARY

As described, mutations activating kinase signaling can now be identified in the majority of patients with LCH and ECD. Although histiocytoses are classified under lymphoid neoplasms in the most recently proposed 2016 WHO classification,[51] increasing gene expression and functional analyses of these disorders suggest that histiocytic neoplasms are closer to the myeloid origin than lymphoid. Thus, reconsideration of the placement of these conditions within the rubric of the 2016 revision of WHO classification is needed. Moreover, discovery of these mutations has led to important therapeutic advances for adults with histiocytosis. Nonetheless, a number of important biological, genetic, and therapeutic questions remain for patients with histiocytoses. First, the precise cell of origin of LCH and ECD remain to be clarified further. Although recent data suggest that *BRAF* V600E mutations may be detected in CD34+ cells in patients with LCH, functional evidence of the disease-initiating capacity of these cells remains to be demonstrated in xenograft studies. Moreover, the cell of origin of non-LCH neoplasms have not been investigated.

From a molecular level, the sustained progress that has been made thus far in understanding the molecular underpinnings of LCH and ECD would now be further propelled by genetic studies focused on specific histologic subsets of histiocytoses such as HS and JXG. Such studies are now needed to better describe, classify, and ultimately treat these forms of histiocytoses whose pathogenesis may differ from that of the more common subtypes. Furthermore, we still do not know the frequency of kinase fusions in patients with histiocytosis. Greater systematic use of RNA-seq analysis to identify fusions will therefore be important moving forward. In addition, the landscape of potentially recurrent genetic events cooperating with kinase mutations in histiocytosis remains to be defined.

Finally, in terms of therapeutic advances, the demonstration of the efficacy of single-agent RAF inhibition as well as preliminary evidence of the efficacy of single-agent MEK inhibition in adults with *BRAF* V600E-mutant histiocytic neoplasms has led to questions of whether RAF, MEK, or combined RAF plus MEK inhibition should be recommended for initial therapy. For those patients lacking the *BRAF* V600E mutation, prospective clinical trial data regarding the usefulness of MEK inhibition is awaited. Moreover, with the application of technology for accurate detection and serial tracking of genetic alterations in plasma cell-free DNA, mutational analysis for histiocytosis-associated somatic mutations in plasma and urine will be very helpful for less invasive and more frequent monitoring of disease activity in patients with ECD/LCH.[52] Finally, further data about the usefulness and safety of targeted therapy against RAF and MEK are needed to make decisions for those children with LCH who are relapsed or refractory to convention, nontargeted therapy.

REFERENCES

1. Hutter C, Kauer M, Simonitsch-Klupp I, et al. Notch is active in Langerhans cell histiocytosis and confers pathognomonic features on dendritic cells. Blood 2012;120(26):5199–208.
2. Allen CE, Li L, Peters TL, et al. Cell-specific gene expression in Langerhans cell histiocytosis lesions reveals a distinct profile compared with epidermal Langerhans cells. J Immunol 2010;184(8):4557–67.
3. Berres ML, Lim KP, Peters T, et al. BRAF-V600E expression in precursor versus differentiated dendritic cells defines clinically distinct LCH risk groups. J Exp Med 2014;211(4):669–83.
4. Swerdlow SH, Campo E, Harris NL, et al. 4th edition. WHO classification of tumours of haematopoietic and lymphoid tissues, vol. 2. WHO Press; 2008.
5. Emile JF, Abla O, Fraitag S, et al. Revised classification of histiocytoses and neoplasms of the macrophage-dendritic cell lineages. Blood 2016;127(22):2672–81.
6. Badalian-Very G, Vergilio JA, Degar BA, et al. Recurrent BRAF mutations in Langerhans cell histiocytosis. Blood 2010;116(11):1919–23.
7. Haroche J, Charlotte F, Arnaud L, et al. High prevalence of BRAF V600E mutations in Erdheim-Chester disease but not in other non-Langerhans cell histiocytoses. Blood 2012;120(13):2700–3.
8. Hervier B, Haroche J, Arnaud L, et al. Association of both Langerhans cell histiocytosis and Erdheim-Chester disease linked to the BRAFV600E mutation. Blood 2014;124(7):1119–26.
9. Go H, Jeon YK, Huh J, et al. Frequent detection of BRAF(V600E) mutations in histiocytic and dendritic cell neoplasms. Histopathology 2014;65(2):261–72.
10. Kansal R, Quintanilla-Martinez L, Datta V, et al. Identification of the V600D mutation in Exon 15 of the BRAF oncogene in congenital, benign Langerhans cell histiocytosis. Genes Chromosomes Cancer 2013;52(1):99–106.
11. Rollins BJ. Genomic alterations in Langerhans cell histiocytosis. Hematol Oncol Clin North Am 2015;29(5):839–51.
12. Kordes M, Röring M, Heining C, et al. Cooperation of BRAF(F595L) and mutant HRAS in histiocytic sarcoma provides new insights into oncogenic BRAF signaling. Leukemia 2016;30(4):937–46.
13. Nakajima Y, Yamada M, Taguchi R, et al. NR4A1 (Nur77) mediates thyrotropin-releasing hormone-induced stimulation of transcription of the thyrotropin beta gene: analysis of TRH knockout mice. PLoS One 2012;7(7):e40437.

14. Chakraborty R, Burke TM, Hampton OA, et al. Alternative genetic mechanisms of BRAF activation in Langerhans cell histiocytosis. Blood 2016;128(21):2533–7.

15. Estep AL, Palmer C, McCormick F, et al. Mutation analysis of BRAF, MEK1 and MEK2 in 15 ovarian cancer cell lines: implications for therapy. PLoS One 2007; 2(12):e1279.

16. Hanrahan AJ, Schultz N, Westfal ML, et al. Genomic complexity and AKT dependence in serous ovarian cancer. Cancer Discov 2012;2(1):56–67.

17. Jeck WR, Parker J, Carson CC, et al. Targeted next generation sequencing identifies clinically actionable mutations in patients with melanoma. Pigment Cell Melanoma Res 2014;27(4):653–63.

18. Brown NA, Furtado LV, Betz BL, et al. High prevalence of somatic MAP2K1 mutations in BRAF V600E-negative Langerhans cell histiocytosis. Blood 2014; 124(10):1655–8.

19. Chakraborty R, Hampton OA, Shen X, et al. Mutually exclusive recurrent somatic mutations in MAP2K1 and BRAF support a central role for ERK activation in LCH pathogenesis. Blood 2014;124(19):3007–15.

20. Nelson DS, Quispel W, Badalian-Very G, et al. Somatic activating ARAF mutations in Langerhans cell histiocytosis. Blood 2014;123(20):3152–5.

21. Diamond EL, Durham BH, Haroche J, et al. Diverse and targetable kinase alterations drive histiocytic neoplasms. Cancer Discov 2016;6(2):154–65.

22. Nelson DS, van Halteren A, Quispel WT, et al. MAP2K1 and MAP3K1 mutations in Langerhans cell histiocytosis. Genes Chromosomes Cancer 2015;54(6):361–8.

23. Chiu A, Ozkaya N, Dogan A. Oncogenic MAP2K1 mutation in a transdifferentiated histiocytic sarcoma. European Association for Haematopathology Meeting. Basel (Switzerland), September 8, 2016. LYWS Case 372. 2016.

24. Emile JF, Diamond EL, Hélias-Rodzewicz Z, et al. Recurrent RAS and PIK3CA mutations in Erdheim-Chester disease. Blood 2014;124(19):3016–9.

25. Ozono S, Inada H, Nakagawa S, et al. Juvenile myelomonocytic leukemia characterized by cutaneous lesion containing Langerhans cell histiocytosis-like cells. Int J Hematol 2011;93(3):389–93.

26. Li Q, Haigis KM, McDaniel A, et al. Hematopoiesis and leukemogenesis in mice expressing oncogenic NrasG12D from the endogenous locus. Blood 2011; 117(6):2022–32.

27. Heritier S, Saffroy R, Radosevic-Robin N, et al. Common cancer-associated PIK3CA activating mutations rarely occur in Langerhans cell histiocytosis. Blood 2015;125(15):2448–9.

28. Brown RA, Kwong BY, McCalmont TH, et al. ETV3-NCOA2 in indeterminate cell histiocytosis: clonal translocation supports sui generis. Blood 2015;126(20): 2344–5.

29. Lee LH, Gasilina A, Roychoudhury J, et al. Real-time genomic profiling of histiocytoses identifies early-kinase domain BRAF alterations while improving treatment outcomes. JCI Insight 2017;2(3):e89473.

30. Takeuchi K, Choi YL, Togashi Y, et al. KIF5B-ALK, a novel fusion oncokinase identified by an immunohistochemistry-based diagnostic system for ALK-positive lung cancer. Clin Cancer Res 2009;15(9):3143–9.

31. Soda M, Choi YL, Enomoto M, et al. Identification of the transforming EML4-ALK fusion gene in non-small-cell lung cancer. Nature 2007;448(7153):561–6.

32. Wiesner T, He J, Yelensky R, et al. Kinase fusions are frequent in Spitz tumours and spitzoid melanomas. Nat Commun 2014;5:3116.

33. Agaram NP, Zhang L, Sung YS, et al. Recurrent NTRK1 gene fusions define a novel subset of locally aggressive lipofibromatosis-like neural tumors. Am J Surg Pathol 2016;40(10):1407–16.

34. Wang L, Motoi T, Khanin R, et al. Identification of a novel, recurrent HEY1-NCOA2 fusion in mesenchymal chondrosarcoma based on a genome-wide screen of exon-level expression data. Genes Chromosomes Cancer 2012;51(2):127–39.

35. Mesquita B, Lopes P, Rodrigues A, et al. Frequent copy number gains at 1q21 and 1q32 are associated with overexpression of the ETS transcription factors ETV3 and ELF3 in breast cancer irrespective of molecular subtypes. Breast Cancer Res Treat 2013;138(1):37–45.

36. Carapeti M, Aguiar RC, Goldman JM, et al. A novel fusion between MOZ and the nuclear receptor coactivator TIF2 in acute myeloid leukemia. Blood 1998;91(9): 3127–33.

37. Deguchi K, Ayton PM, Carapeti M, et al. MOZ-TIF2-induced acute myeloid leukemia requires the MOZ nucleosome binding motif and TIF2-mediated recruitment of CBP. Cancer Cell 2003;3(3):259–71.

38. Strehl S, Nebral K, König M, et al. ETV6-NCOA2: a novel fusion gene in acute leukemia associated with coexpression of T-lymphoid and myeloid markers and frequent NOTCH1 mutations. Clin Cancer Res 2008;14(4):977–83.

39. Sumegi J, Streblow R, Frayer RW, et al. Recurrent t(2;2) and t(2;8) translocations in rhabdomyosarcoma without the canonical PAX-FOXO1 fuse PAX3 to members of the nuclear receptor transcriptional coactivator family. Genes Chromosomes Cancer 2010;49(3):224–36.

40. Hyman DM, Puzanov I, Subbiah V, et al. Vemurafenib in Multiple Nonmelanoma Cancers with BRAF V600 Mutations. N Engl J Med 2015;373(8):726–36.

41. Diamond EL, Subbiah V, Lockhart C, et al. Vemurafenib in Patients with Erdheim–Chester Disease (ECD) and Langerhans Cell Histiocytosis (LCH) Harboring BRAFV600 Mutations: A Cohort of the Histology-Independent VE-Basket Study. Blood 128(22);480.

42. Haroche J, Cohen-Aubart F, Emile JF, et al. Reproducible and sustained efficacy of targeted therapy with vemurafenib in patients with BRAF(V600E)-mutated Erdheim-Chester disease. J Clin Oncol 2015;33(5):411–8.

43. Kieran MW, Hargrave DR, Cohen KJ, et al. Phase 1 study of dabrafenib in pediatric patients (pts) with relapsed or refractory BRAF V600E high- and low-grade gliomas (HGG, LGG), Langerhans cell histiocytosis (LCH), and other solid tumors (OST). J Clin Oncol 2015;33(suppl; abstr 10004).

44. Nordmann TM, Juengling FD, Recher M, et al. Trametinib after disease reactivation under dabrafenib in Erdheim-Chester disease with both BRAF and KRAS mutations. Blood 2017;129(7):879–82.

45. Cohen Aubart F, Emile JF, Maksud P, et al. Efficacy of the MEK inhibitor cobimetinib for wild-type BRAF Erdheim-Chester disease. Br J Haematol 2016. [Epub ahead of print].

46. Emery CM, Vijayendran KG, Zipser MC, et al. MEK1 mutations confer resistance to MEK and B-RAF inhibition. Proc Natl Acad Sci U S A 2009;106(48):20411–6.

47. Azorsa D, Lee DW, Bista R, et al. Association of clinical and biological resistance with a novel mutation in MAP2K1 in a patient with Langerhans cell histiocytosis. J Clin Oncol 2016;34 (2016 ASCO) Abstract.

48. Diamond EL, Durham BH, Dogan A, et al. Phase 2 Trial of Single-Agent Cobimetinib for Adults with Histiocytic Disorders: Preliminary Results (abstract). 2016 Erdheim Chester Disease Global Alliance Medical Symposium.

49. Larkin J, Ascierto PA, Dréno B, et al. Combined vemurafenib and cobimetinib in BRAF-mutated melanoma. N Engl J Med 2014;371(20):1867–76.
50. Gianfreda D, Nicastro M, Galetti M, et al. Sirolimus plus prednisone for Erdheim-Chester disease: an open-label trial. Blood 2015;126(10):1163–71.
51. Swerdlow SH, Campo E, Pileri SA, et al. The 2016 revision of the World Health Organization classification of lymphoid neoplasms. Blood 2016;127(20):2375–90.
52. Hyman DM, Diamond EL, Vibat CR, et al. Prospective blinded study of BRAFV600E mutation detection in cell-free DNA of patients with systemic histio-cytic disorders. Cancer Discov 2015;5(1):64–71.

Moving?

Make sure your subscription moves with you!

To notify us of your new address, find your **Clinics Account Number** (located on your mailing label above your name), and contact customer service at:

Email: journalscustomerservice-usa@elsevier.com

800-654-2452 (subscribers in the U.S. & Canada)
314-447-8871 (subscribers outside of the U.S. & Canada)

Fax number: 314-447-8029

Elsevier Health Sciences Division
Subscription Customer Service
3251 Riverport Lane
Maryland Heights, MO 63043

*To ensure uninterrupted delivery of your subscription, please notify us at least 4 weeks in advance of move.

Printed and bound by CPI Group (UK) Ltd, Croydon, CR0 4YY

03/10/2024

01040395-0017